meditations

FOR

PAIN
RECOVERY

BY

TONY GRECO

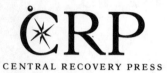

CENTRAL RECOVERY PRESS

CENTRAL RECOVERY PRESS

Central Recovery Press (CRP) is committed to publishing exceptional materials addressing addiction treatment, recovery, and behavioral health care, including original and quality books, audio/visual communications, and Web-based new media. Through a diverse selection of titles, it seeks to impact the behavioral health care field with a broad range of unique resources for professionals, recovering individuals and their families, and the general public.

For more information, visit www.centralrecoverypress.com.

Central Recovery Press, Las Vegas, NV 89129
© 2010 by Central Recovery Press, Las Vegas, NV

ISBN-13: 978-0-9818482-8-0
ISBN-10: 0-9818482-8-1

All rights reserved. Published 2010. Printed in the United States of America.

16 15 14 13 12 11 10   1 2 3 4 5

Publisher: Central Recovery Press
            3371 N Buffalo Drive
            Las Vegas, NV 89129

Cover design and interior by Sara Streifel, Think Creative Design
Photo of Tony Greco by Russell Persky

{ ACKNOWLEDGMENTS }

*Thanks to the staff of the Las Vegas Recovery Center
and Central Recovery Press for all their help
in the creation of this book.*

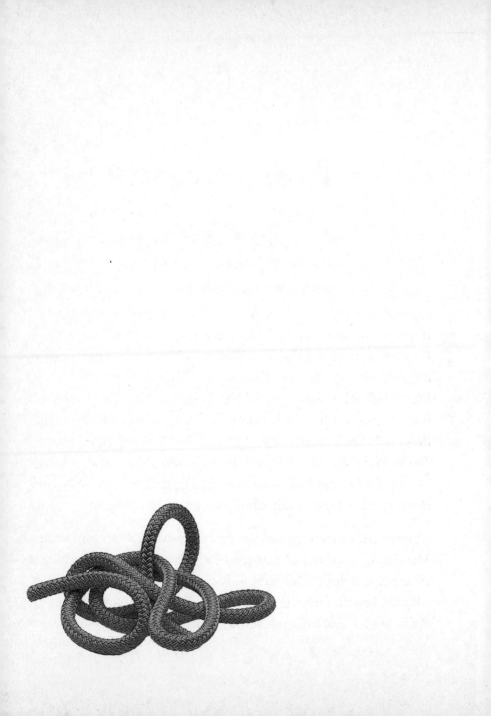

{ INTRODUCTION }

Meditations for Pain Recovery is designed for people suffering from chronic pain and recovering from addiction to pain medication. It is a companion book to A *Day without Pain* by Mel Pohl, MD, FASAM, with Mike Donohue; *Pain Recovery: How to Find Balance and Reduce Suffering from Chronic Pain* by Mel Pohl, MD, FASAM, Frank J. Szabo, Jr., LADC, Daniel Shiode, Ph.D., and Robert Hunter, Ph.D.; and *Pain Recovery for Families: How to Find Balance When Someone Else's Chronic Pain Becomes Your Problem Too* by Mel Pohl, MD, FASAM, Frank J. Szabo, Jr., LADC, Daniel Shiode, Ph.D., and Robert Hunter, Ph.D. However, this book can also be read independently of any other book or program.

Chronic pain affects approximately seventy-two million Americans. The risks of using opioid pain medication and developing addiction are explained thoroughly in *Pain Recovery*. You need not be an addict to benefit from these daily meditations; however, the premise of this book is that the reader is abstinent from opioids and other mind- and/or mood-altering chemicals. There is also an assumption that those using this meditation book are active in a recovery process and have a therapist, sponsor, or counselor, as well as a support group, whether formal or informal, therapeutic, and/or twelve-step-based.

Each meditation in this book is based on one of five categories taken from either the "four points of balance" or material on relationships in recovery, which are explained in detail in the book *Pain Recovery*, along with a reflection for each. According to *Pain Recovery*, "The four points of balance are applicable to any situation in life, including chronic pain." Use what works for you and leave the rest.

More on the Four Points of Balance and Relationships from the Book *Pain Recovery*:

PHYSICAL BALANCE

Physical balance meditations will call attention to your being mindful and respectful of your body on a given day. These meditations will guide you to pay attention to the messages your body sends to your brain. On these days you will be guided to evaluate the state of your body thoroughly and continually, although you will do so without becoming preoccupied, asking questions such as:

✆ How am I feeling?

✆ If there is pain, where is it coming from and how bad is it?

- What action that has worked in the past might I take to modify it—stretch, change position, get up and move, breathe, listen to soothing music, talk to someone (reach out), or share with someone who is also hurting (give back)?

On days of physical balance, you may be directed to the organized series of maintenance and crisis interventions in the book *Pain Recovery* that includes regular exercise, meditation, massage, stretching, and chiropractic treatments, in addition to other balancing actions.

Characteristics of a balanced physical experience are:

- Eating nutritious foods
- Avoiding toxins
- Exercising regularly
- Getting enough sleep
- Practicing relaxation

MENTAL BALANCE

Mental balance meditations will challenge the assumptions you have about your pain and the thought processes surrounding your recovery. Your pain is neither the worst that ever existed nor is it insignificant. It is not a punishment; it is simply an occurrence in the course of your life that has various challenging ripple effects. Balanced thinking results in creating a realistic set of goals and focusing energy and effort into making progress toward achieving each one. This progress leads to diminishment of pain, decreased suffering, and increased function, empowering you to set new goals and work toward achieving them. On mental balance days, pain recovery is based not on blind faith, but on well-thought-out, realistic expectations, and on progressive success that is achieved by applying the tools you have learned in pain recovery. During these days you will continue to see how you change or do not change your thought patterns, and practice using the tools you acquire. Characteristics of mental balance are:

- Keeping a positive attitude
- Paying attention to and challenging your thoughts
- Setting achievable goals
- Being open-minded and willing to try new things
- Having realistic hope

EMOTIONAL BALANCE

With emotional balance, you accept your emotions and know that it's okay to feel what you are feeling. On days focused on emotional balance you will continue to remind yourself that you need not be focused on the opinions of others, but that you can focus on hearing and trusting in your own inner voice. You identify your feelings and recognize that they are a major part of you that should be honored. You accept who you are and what you feel in the present moment, and that acceptance allows you to continue making positive changes in your life. Accepting your feelings and being emotionally balanced keeps you from feeling recurring negative emotions. With a focus on emotional balance every few days, you will continue to feel your full emotional experience, knowing that all of your feelings are a part of you. When you are emotionally balanced you are continuing to work toward resolving old issues that you had once avoided, and you work to heal and release your connection to the past, allowing yourself to be free to live in the moment. You are able to feel emotions for each circumstance that shows up in your life without troublesome attachment to old feelings. Characteristics of emotional balance are:

- Understanding that feelings are neither good nor bad
- Understanding that experiencing feelings will not hurt you
- Knowing that feeling your feelings results in healing
- Realizing that balanced thoughts create balanced emotions

SPIRITUAL BALANCE

Spiritual balance consists of being connected to your thoughts and feelings and the way you care for your body. When balanced, your spirituality enhances your life. You do positive things that make you feel good, and you help others. You are in harmony with the world and those in it. Whatever life brings, you are able to deal with it and know you are okay. You are able to find meaning and purpose even in situations that are painful. You live in and accept each day as it comes, changing yourself instead of trying to change others. Characteristics of spiritual balance include:

- Accepting who you are
- Having a sense of purpose
- Being open to changing beliefs
- Drawing on a source of inner and outer strength

- Having values, beliefs, standards, and ethics
- Being aware and appreciative of a "transcendent dimension" to life beyond you
- Having increased awareness of a connection to self, others, God/Spirit/Divine, and nature through regular spiritual practices

RELATIONSHIPS

Relationships have a category of their own in *Meditations for Pain Recovery*, because like everyone on earth, you have numerous types of relationships, such as:

- Social
- Intimate
- Acquaintanceship

- Familial
- Romantic
- Business

All of these relationships affect and are affected by your experience of chronic pain. Your relationships are not only an outward manifestation and indication of your overall state of balance; they also have an effect on your state of balance, either negatively or positively.

As you read and think about the meditations in this book each day, it is my hope that you will take ownership of your pain recovery on a daily basis.

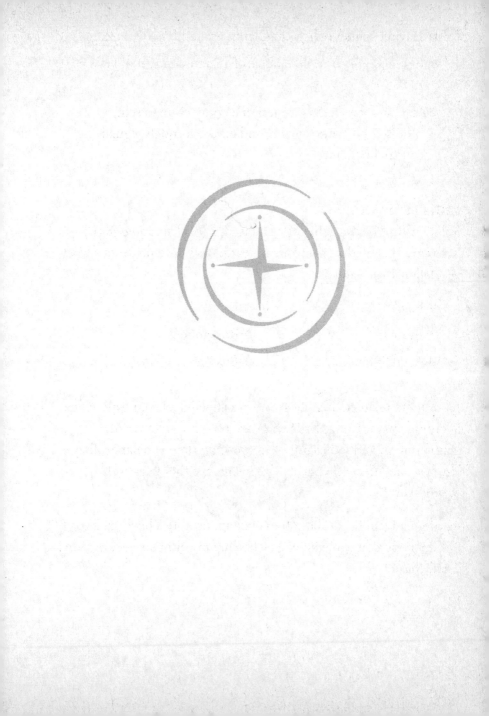

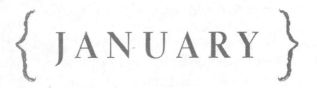

{ JANUARY }

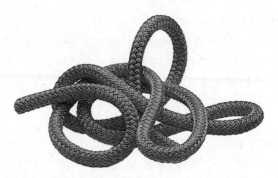

NEW BEGINNINGS

THE FOUR POINTS OF BALANCE

"It is better to spend one day contemplating the birth
and death of all things than a hundred years never
contemplating beginnings and endings."
Siddhartha Gautama, the Buddha

Today is a new beginning for me, and I want to take a moment
to contemplate what that means.

The four points of balance are physical, mental, emotional, and
spiritual—and today I am learning new tools and techniques to help
me with each one of these elements of my life and my recovery. As
I begin this book of meditations for pain recovery, I'm aware that
I don't expect to become pain-free—my expectations are that if I
apply the tools of my program of recovery to each of the points of
balance, my life can be restored to a manageable state of sanity,
provided I do the work. With the help of my higher power, may
this new beginning be an auspicious one.

*I'm addressing my thoughts, feelings, spirituality, relationships, and
behaviors in a new way today; without abusing pain medications, I am
changing my relationship with myself and my physical pain.*

AMENDS

PHYSICAL BALANCE

"Making amends in recovery is not
simply saying, 'I'm sorry.'"
Tails of Recovery: Addicts and the Pets That Love Them

In the past, I harmed my body through my dependence on pain medication, so today I make a living amend to my body by treating my pain in healthy ways—by moving and exercising instead of self-medicating and wanting to be catered to or babied.

In active addiction, I neglected my body by abusing medication rather than turning to physical activity. Today I live my amends to my body, mind, and spirit even on the many days when I do not feel like making myself exercise, move, or even get out of bed. Sometimes it seems downright mean to my body to force it to move because of the physical pain I am experiencing, but I remember the alternative of being addicted to pain medication. Today I know that pain recovery requires me to keep moving.

I make amends to myself by continuing my physical routine. I know that even when it does not feel like it, it is the most loving thing to do.

MOVEMENT

MENTAL BALANCE

....

"It has been shown that when the minds of people
in pain were distracted by something that required
intense concentration, their brain's pain centers
demonstrated decreased activity."
A Day without Pain

I can't sit around and say I'll do something once I'm feeling better,
because sitting around waiting to feel better is self-defeating.
Actually doing something is what helps me feel better…it's a case
of "bring the body and the mind follows."

When my mind and body are in activity, in movement, in the
solution, I'm able to bring my spirit into balance with them.
Through movement, my mind is better able to focus on that
which is the real solution to most of my problems: a loving, caring,
connected relationship with my higher self and higher power.
Through this connection, I help my mind slow down, and the mind
slowing helps my body slow down, thus decreasing my pain. The
cycle is continuous, always affecting the next thing, a flow, so to
speak, or a spiral that is either going up into the light or down into
the darkness. I move along this spiral; I dance along the balance
of mind-body-spirit, affecting one, affecting all.

*When I'm feeling stuck, I unstick myself by moving—first, by moving
my body, which moves my mind, and thereby moves my spirit. My
spirit in balance can then better hold my body in love rather than
my body holding my spirit in pain.*

COURAGE

EMOTIONAL BALANCE

....

"In recovery, we begin to know courage by watching
and respecting others who tell us they are afraid and
then find the spiritual and emotional resources to walk
through their fear to do the right thing."
Of Character: Building Assets in Recovery

Walking through pain, fear, shame, guilt, loneliness, and anger
without heading down a path of destruction is the goal in recovery.
These are all feelings that, in moderation, are necessary and vital to
the human experience. The problem with addiction is the extreme
to which I feel these feelings. The problem with chronic pain is the
lack of tolerance I have for any other feelings beyond the physical
pain. When all my energy and resources are being dedicated to
that single source of one kind of pain, it feels impossible to deal
with anything else, and if I let it, a small thing may become the
proverbial straw that breaks the camel's back. It takes a special kind
of courage to live free from active addiction. It takes a leap of what
can seem like superhuman strength and courage to live free from
addiction and with chronic pain. This courage may not start within,
but that's where it leads. The path to courage is paved with steps,
sponsors, meetings, prayer, and meditation.

*When I'm feeling discouraged, I act on courage; I go the extra distance,
with an added result of developing more strength and a closer, deeper
relationship with my higher power.*

PEACE

SPIRITUAL BALANCE

"Music is the silence between the notes."
Claude Debussy

If it's true that the silence between the notes creates music, then perhaps the periods when I feel my pain create the periods of peace I also enjoy. All human beings deal with pain. The contrast between the high and the low—pain and no pain or less pain—is what helps me appreciate the music of my life. It's easy to just focus on the pain, but I must remember to focus on the peace in between the pain.

Pain lets me know I am alive. At times I may not be prepared to feel my pain, but I know its existence serves a necessary purpose. My automatic reactions and my emotional state affect how I feel my pain. If I can change my reactions and learn to identify and accept my emotions, pain will continue to serve its proper purpose.

I must accept my pain, but it must not become my master. Pain can be part of my life, but I cannot allow it to become my whole existence. My pain can motivate me to help others who suffer. When I help others, the voice of my pain becomes fainter. Its whisper, however, remains a part of my very being.

Pain is like a rainy day; although it can bring me sadness, rain is necessary in order to nourish and nurture the flowers that bring me joy. So does my pain nourish my spirit, even though it too brings sadness; however, it makes my experience of life complete. I embrace my pain and continue to seek the many colors of life's rainbow.

ADVERSITY

RELATIONSHIPS

....

"Sweet are the uses of adversity, which, like a toad, though ugly and venomous, wears yet a precious jewel in its head."
William Shakespeare

It is much easier for me to do the things I need to do for my recovery when things are going my way. It's easy to be an angel when no one is ruffling my feathers. During a regular day I take some comfort in my routine of waking up in the morning, praying and meditating, doing my physical exercises, going to work, attending my recovery meeting, and having a relaxing evening at home. Then trouble strikes.

Maybe my pain is extraordinarily bad, the kids are acting up, my partner is not "behaving" the way I'd like, or there are problems at work. Any one of those situations can create problems in any other, and I am faced with adversity in my life. My natural response is to break the healthy habits in my life and fall back on old habits: crying out from my pain, not feeling well enough to exercise, calling in sick to work, or not feeling like I have enough energy or strength to make it to a meeting. During my struggles in relationships it is more important than ever to reinforce the healthy habits in my life and not fall back on old habits that created far more adversity in my life than anything going on today.

I focus on the new habits in my life regardless of the adversity in my life. The routine and habits I establish in my recovery are not negotiable. My life and my relationships depend on these good habits, and no amount of adversity in my life is made better by falling back into old routines.

APPRECIATION

PHYSICAL BALANCE

....

*"If you can't appreciate what you have got,
then get what you appreciate."*
Unknown

When is the last time I did something nice for myself? Have
I taken myself to the spa lately? Have I gotten a pedicure or
manicure? Maybe it is time for a massage. In pain recovery I learn
to be appreciative of my body and the things it can do, rather than
focusing on the things it cannot do. But do I actually show that
appreciation? I run myself around, work hard, and work through
my pain, but all too often it's easy to let a whole day go by without
having physical appreciation for what I have. I can do this in the
simplest of ways: just massaging my feet, getting a nice lotion to rub
on my arms and legs, taking a warm bath, or getting into the hot
tub. In whatever way I choose—and it may be something I do
every day, anyway—I do it with the intention of showing my
body that I appreciate it.

*I show my body appreciation by doing something special for it today.
In doing things I normally do anyway, I make sure my intention is
dedicated and focused on appreciation for my body and physically
showing that body how grateful I am.*

MEMORY

MENTAL BALANCE

---

*"His heart was as great as the world, but there was
no room in it to hold the memory of a wrong."*
Ralph Waldo Emerson

My body not only remembers past injuries and significant changes
in its structure and function, but it also holds onto past experiences.
While my mind is quick to notice when my body is reminding me of
physical trauma, my mind does not necessarily comprehend when
my body is reminding me of other traumas. My mind may have
blocked out certain experiences and memories for a reason. Perhaps
my conscious mind is not ready to remember, so my body holds and
stores the memory until I'm ready to address it. As a result, I may feel
pain in different places where I had no physical injury.

The more I recover, the more my body is free from focusing
on the area of chronic pain and is freed to start releasing pains
and memories in other places. Without abusing medication and
through working the steps, my body is starting to tell my mind that
it is time to take these memories, process them, and be free from
them. My mind cooperates with my body to work through my pain.

*I reveal, heal, and instill new physical memories in my body by
focusing my mind on the continuing journey of pain recovery. My
body begins to release old and painful memories because my mind can
handle it. In pain recovery, I catch those memories and release them to
the love and light so that healing can happen in every area.*

APPRECIATION

EMOTIONAL BALANCE

....

*"Appreciation is a wonderful thing. It makes what
is excellent in others belong to us as well."*
Voltaire

A balanced life may at times seem elusive. Just when I feel like things are going smoothly, I encounter a bump in the road. Recovery, just like life, is full of moments such as this. One of the many gifts I've received in recovery is a conscious awareness of myself that includes my actions, behaviors, and relationships with others. This ability doesn't come naturally—it is something I must train myself to acknowledge physically, mentally, emotionally, and spiritually.

This process takes place minute by minute and day by day. It is when I experience moments of physical pain that I must reach within and put to use all of the tools that are available. It is my goal to practice awareness, tolerance, and acceptance for those things that are out of my control. Chronic pain isn't something that can be controlled, but the way I view my pain can be.

I am patient with myself and accept those things over which I have no control. In addition, I do my part in identifying what I can manage, and look to my higher power, sponsor, and support group for strength, direction, and encouragement. I don't have to do this alone. When I acknowledge and accept this, I move further into appreciation and gratitude, which then transcends into love for myself.

RECOVERY

SPIRITUAL BALANCE

"Recovery gives us a road back to health
and true living, but it is rarely easy."
Tails of Recovery: Addicts and the Pets That Love Them

"I'm different." When I was new in recovery, I felt different
because my family had no history of addiction, and yet I had
become dependent on my medication to manage a "legitimate"
chronic pain condition. I was appalled to consider that I was
addicted—surely I was nothing like the stereotypical addict
in movies or on television! Was I?

Yes! That was certainly not an easy thing to accept. And yet,
when I did come to realize and accept that my dependence was
just like that of any other addict, I learned to grow spiritually. When
I see the similarities between myself and others in recovery, my
spirituality can flourish. It's not always easy to look at the
truth about myself, but any life in recovery is much easier than
a life in active addiction.

*I seek identification with the recovery process and don't waste energy
trying to find ways that the principles of recovery don't apply to me.
Doing that only keeps me in the self-imposed prison of addiction and
pain. Today, I take comfort in the fact that I am not unique in recovery.*

GETTING INTO THE SOLUTION, POSITIVE ACTION

RELATIONSHIPS

"My recovery is solution-based, and I apply principles of the Twelve Steps in the context of chronic pain in all of my relationships. My goal is to stop feeling like a victim of my pain and instead to live in acceptance and hope, have a positive attitude, and take positive action with regard to others. I have taken a huge step in healing my relationships and continue to do so daily by remembering my powerlessness over chronic pain."

Adapted from Pain Recovery: How to Find Balance and Reduce Suffering from Chronic Pain

Positive action allows me to open up on new levels, receiving the life-changing gifts of recovery. I give back to others what I have been given so freely. It takes willingness and effort, but my recovery is worth it to me.

Recovery and living in the solution is an ongoing process that requires looking honestly at myself, continuing to be open-minded to new solutions and new tools as I face new challenges in my life without abusing pain medication.

ATTITUDE

PHYSICAL BALANCE

Human beings, by changing the inner attitudes of their
minds, can change the outer aspects of their lives.
William James

My attitude can and does affect my physical health, well-being,
and life balance. I discovered this from the very beginning of
recovery, when I was first trying to live without the use of addictive
medications to help me through my day. I realized that my pain
and the way it affected the other areas of my own health were often
the result of the attitude that I had about life and my pain.
By shifting my attitude I have the ability to actually improve
my own health.

When I am not feeling well, whether as a result of my pain or
simply because of a cold or flu, I have the ability to make things
better or worse for myself based on my attitude. If I happen to be
sick on a given day and cannot or should not go to work, I can
either be depressed and obsess about this feeling too much—just
like my old behavior—or I can use the time to get caught up on
reading something that will inspire me in my recovery.

*My attitude affects my health and physical balance. I remember that
a positive attitude results in my feeling and being healthier.*

LOVE

MENTAL BALANCE

"You, yourself, as much as anybody in the entire
universe, deserve your love and affection."
Siddhartha Gautama, the Buddha

Love has many faces: love of family, love of a partner, love of
country, love of life. And all of these can start with a healthy love
of self. Loving myself means treating myself differently today; I do
what I need to stay healthy and strong—that's self-love, and it is
the foundation of all other loves in my life.

Love is one of the highest vibrations of energy I can use, a healing
energy that has the power to do what no medication, no other
behavior, person, place, or thing ever could. By shifting my mind-
state into a state of love, I can change the way I feel, think, and act
in life, thus changing the response of those around me, my relation
to them, and my effect on them and them on me. I can think of
myself and of others with love, and love is what I get in return.

*I love being alive and in my body, I love my higher power, and
that power loves me. With love at the forefront of my mind, I can use
that energy to be in this body, be present-centered, and let go of
past hurts, wrongs, and pain.*

RESPONSIBILITY

EMOTIONAL BALANCE

....

*"Learning they are not responsible for their disease, but
that they must be responsible for learning how to live
life without drugs, is, without question, a big challenge
for most addicts to face in recovery."*
Tails of Recovery: Addicts and the Pets That Love Them

My addiction to pain medication caused my life to spiral out of
control emotionally. I was taking more than was prescribed because
the medication seemed to have stopped working. I began taking
more and more to cover up the emotional pain that came as a result
of the medication not managing my chronic pain. I was constantly
lying to myself and others about how much medication I
was taking. I was ashamed of myself.

Eventually I hit bottom and had to take responsibility, not only for
how much I was using and abusing, but for why I was using and
abusing. It was not necessarily because of the physical chronic pain
anymore. Using had become my way to handle life on its terms as
a result of having pain. It was a natural progression that happens
to many people. Taking responsibility means not making excuses
anymore. Taking responsibility means accepting all the feelings —
good and bad — that are attached to what happened to me.

*Taking responsibility means my life is different today. I am
clean and in recovery. I do not judge myself by what I did in my
addiction; instead I take responsibility for my actions and continue
to work on my recovery.*

.

SERVICE

SPIRITUAL BALANCE

....

"It is one of the most beautiful compensations
of this life that no man can sincerely try to help
another without helping himself."
Ralph Waldo Emerson

One of the keys to twelve-step recovery, regardless of the
manifestation of addiction, is service. Ultimately, all of the steps lead
to the inevitable end of carrying the message of recovery to another
person who is still suffering. I do not need to wait until I have formally
worked a Twelfth Step with a sponsor in order to practice this
principle. In fact, I may not ever get the opportunity to work a Twelfth
Step if I do not start practicing this principle as soon as possible.

I ask my higher power to use me to help any of his children who
need help, whether they are "old" or new in recovery.

When I'm feeling that my chronic pain is too much for me to
bear, I get out of myself and find a spiritual connection with a
higher power by connecting with another person who needs help.
I can be of service to this person, sharing, listening, or just being
present, and I find my higher power through that connection. Once
connected to my higher power, I'm disconnected from the
intensity and power of my chronic pain.

*Trusting in the recovery process can teach me that I can manage my pain
without using substances. Having had this experience, I can more effectively
help others who are trying to recover, as the Twelfth Step instructs.*

BEING NONJUDGMENTAL

RELATIONSHIPS

"How much easier it is to be critical than to be correct."
Benjamin Disraeli

My pain can make me very judgmental toward others if I allow it to. Having judgments against others is a way of putting my own expectations upon them, instead of accepting them as they are. If a person does not behave, speak, or think the way I believe they should, then perhaps there are flaws inside myself that I need to take a closer look at.

I cannot expect others to instinctively know how my pain is affecting me at any given moment. People I may judge as simply insensitive to my pain may be going through problems of their own—and what a wonderful opportunity that might be for me to get outside myself and help them. But if I'm too busy judging them, I miss it.

By being nonjudgmental, and by accepting others as they are instead of expecting them to fulfill my needs, I have an easier time in recovery from both my addiction and my chronic pain.

Judging others makes my pain worse. Pain recovery is being free from judging others and instead practicing acceptance and love.

CRISIS INTERVENTION

PHYSICAL BALANCE

"Luck is what happens
when preparation meets opportunity."
Seneca

When I read *Pain Recovery*, I made a "crisis intervention plan" for times when my pain would become seemingly intolerable. This plan was based on who I was when I first entered recovery, but this plan, like the rest of my recovery, is constantly evolving.

If I have a flare-up of pain today, what is the best course of action for me to take? When I first made my crisis intervention plan, I might not have been able to walk one hundred feet, let alone the mile I may perhaps be in the habit of walking today.

I am prepared for such good and not-so-good days, because with chronic pain those not-so-good days will certainly come. I can be in the habit of certain exercises, but on "bad" days, it's best for me to know what exacerbates the pain and what helps me deal with the pain. Perhaps it may hurt that day to walk, but it might be the best thing for me. It's best to know in advance, with a crisis intervention plan.

I make sure my crisis intervention plan is current. I am prepared for how and what I can do physically when I have a flare-up of pain. I am ready when the time comes, so I know exactly what to do, rather than letting the pain decide what I'll do that day.

LACK OF FOCUS

MENTAL BALANCE

....

"Little by little does the trick."
Aesop

Painful experiences such as job loss, financial difficulties, and legal problems can cause me to be mixed up and lack focus. When I'm in this state it creates physical difficulties. My head aches. My body weakens. Depression sets in, brought about by stress. The final result is increased pain.

I reduce my stress by doing the next right thing. I avoid procrastinating, knowing that "procrastination is the thief of time."

When I'm mixed up and don't know what to focus on next, I focus on my recovery. I take positive action by doing the next right thing, writing about my recovery or taking a moment to read recovery literature. I make sure I've called my sponsor. Then I focus on one thing that needs to be done, be it paying a particular bill, balancing my checkbook, or taking out the trash. Prayer helps focus my mind to help me accomplish the next right task in front of me, thus reducing my stress. Reduced stress—a simplified plan of action, one step at a time—improves my health and reduces my pain.

I regain focus and sort through my mixed-up thoughts and feelings as well as simplify my life by taking care of the small things that need to be done that are directly in front of me. I owe it to myself to try to lead a stress-free life. By taking care of the little everyday things that need to be done, I can focus on what's important: my recovery.

SERVICE

EMOTIONAL BALANCE

"The greatest good you can do for another is not just
to share your riches, but to reveal to him his own."
Benjamin Disraeli

The emotional pain I experience can help me grow. I achieve emotional balance by walking through this pain, and one of the ways I have learned to do this is through service to others. Service takes my focus off myself and my pain, and puts my focus on helping someone else. Working with another person often helps both of us experience the "riches" of recovery.

Through service work, I achieve balance in other areas of my life, and this helps with my chronic pain. Being of service helps me tremendously in all areas of my life, but particularly when I feel like I'm suffering from emotions that come up when actively working a pain recovery program.

Whether at a twelve-step meeting, with my support group, in the community, or in other ways that I discover through working with my counselor, sponsor, or therapist, I am of service to others today.

TOLERANCE

SPIRITUAL BALANCE

"Tolerance has helped me calmly surrender my
need to control people and/or situations. It allows
me to step back, clear my head, and get a better
perspective without going into the over-the-top
dramas I tend to create in my mind."

Tails of Recovery: Addicts and the Pets That Love Them

In active addiction, I could tolerate nothing without abusing
pain medication. Before I knew it, I had turned a useful tool
(medication) into a tool of destruction, because I believed I needed
it to cope with my life and my pain. Then I entered recovery, and
as my head cleared, I realized that in the process of trying to fix my
chronic pain I had broken my ability to handle life on life's terms.

One indispensible ingredient of a life of peace and harmony
is an acceptance, or a tolerance for, all the feelings I experience
on any given day. I embrace multiple feelings, and am able to do
this through an increased spiritual connection with a power greater
than myself. Left to my own devices I cannot tolerate anything,
but with the help of a loving higher power I can tolerate
all that life has to offer.

*I build my tolerance for all my feelings by continually focusing on
my relationship with a higher power. I set myself expectations that I
am able to reach. I do not set myself up for failure. Instead, I try to set
myself up for success. Having faith that my pain is tolerable for the day
allows me to focus on my recovery.*

HONESTY

RELATIONSHIPS

....

A lie is really just a timesaving device, and if it
makes me look better than the truth would, so much
the better. If it gets me whatever I want and helps me
avoid some unpleasant reality, that's best of all.
At least that's what I used to think.

The Soul Workout: Getting and Staying Spiritually Fit

There are lies of commission, and lies of omission. When I don't tell you how much I need your help, that's a lie of omission. That's dishonest.

Today I am honest about my needs, my limitations, my expectations, and my capabilities. I do what I can do today, to the best of my ability, but I ask for help when a task is beyond me. When I was in active addiction, instead of allowing others to help me, I would take on tasks even though I knew they would overwhelm me, because I did not want to appear weak.

I am learning that to ask for help is not a sign of weakness. In the process of being honest in my relationships, I open up to the possibility of getting help from others. I give others the opportunity to be of service. I focus on being honest about my physical limitations, knowing today that they do not make me weak. Not being honest about them does.

I am honest with someone today about my physical pain, what I may need help with, and how I'm feeling. In doing so, I give those around me the power and the choice to help me or not, but I let go of the results and focus only on being honest.

COMPASSION

PHYSICAL BALANCE

"I would rather feel compassion
than know the meaning of it."
Thomas Aquinas

It is important to remember that many with chronic pain have an altered body image. I'm no different. But I don't limit myself with the label "disabled." My focus is no longer on my chronic pain and what I can't do, but on having compassion for others and for myself. Compassion allows me to focus on what I *can* do, for others and for myself. And the more compassion I feel, the more I live in the light of recovery, instead of in the darkness and depression of my disease.

I have compassion for my body and focus on what I can do, rather than focusing on my chronic pain and what I can't do. I remember that I have made huge strides and continue to work on increasing my abilities. I have compassion and love for my body today.

23

KINDNESS

MENTAL BALANCE

"Kindness is in our power,
even when fondness is not."
Samuel Johnson

I gently turn my thoughts to acceptance of physical, mental, emotional, and spiritual limitations, not only in others, but in myself as well. Lack of loving kindness, whether toward others or myself, aggravates my chronic pain. When I'm in pain—be it chronic, acute, or emotional—I channel my thoughts toward asking, without judgment, "Was the pain avoidable?" If I'm responsible, I think about what part, if any, I had in the flare-up or onset of pain. I do this with the intention of using my mind as a tool to show myself kindness by finding and exploring alternative ways to avoid inflicting pain on myself or others in the future.

I am kind to myself and others, and do not allow negative thoughts about myself to slow my growth in recovery. I treat myself with kindness by directing my thoughts to the solution, giving myself permission to live life to the fullest.

MEDITATIONS FOR PAIN RECOVERY | 31

PRAYER

EMOTIONAL BALANCE

....

"Prayer does not change God,
but it changes him who prays."
Søren Kierkegaard

I needed a change in my life when I entered pain recovery.
Prayer has been one of the greatest tools for providing that change,
and it's one that my program of pain recovery has provided me.
When I am emotionally unbalanced, stuck in running "what if"
scenarios repeatedly in my head, or thinking the worst about my
current situation, I must remember that my higher power is as
close as a prayer. I ask my higher power to direct my attention to
His will for me, and away from my painful, destructive, or negative
thoughts. I am no use to myself or to my fellows if I am emotionally
unbalanced. Fortunately, prayer can help me regain the
emotional balance I need for my recovery.

*When I find I'm thinking about the future, running scenarios about
"what if" something happens, I replace those thoughts with a repeated,
internal prayer to ask my higher power for help. I seek out this power to
keep me safe in the moment, as I attempt to feel the emotions I used to
try to avoid in the here and now by thinking about the future.*

COMMITMENT
SPIRITUAL BALANCE

"Being committed requires the consistency
and fortitude to do what is required
even when we are tired or don't feel we can."
Of Character: Building Assets in Recovery

The hidden agenda of every addict is to use. With that in mind,
spirituality requires eternal vigilance. Even when I'm doing my
best, or during the best of times, I have a thought process that is
constantly calculating ways I can find something outside myself to
"fix me" quickly. I seek out instant gratification. I fantasize about
easier, softer (but ultimately more painful) ways and means of being
in the world and dealing with my chronic pain. I must make a
commitment to my pain recovery on a regular, sometimes moment-
by-moment basis. I must constantly monitor all of the points of
balance in my life and at the same time, give myself a break and
take it easy on myself. My commitment is not to be perfect. My
commitment is to being imperfect, but recovering. Recovery is
a process, a journey, and a life of ongoing monitoring, forever
discovering ways I interact with the world.

*I make a commitment to myself and to my higher power that for
this day I will focus on my recovery and not on my pain.*

CONTROL

RELATIONSHIPS

....

"Men are rich only as they give.
He who gives great service gets great rewards."
Elbert Hubbard

Part of active addiction is a belief that I always have to be in
control. In my mind, people who were not in control were people
who were weak. It was one thing to feel disabled by chronic pain,
another thing to be controlled by drugs. My pain has changed the
way I view the world. In my worst moments of pain, I realized I had
no control, and I felt like a victim. When I made that realization
deep in my heart, I became free. I do not feel such a need to
control anymore. Ironically, by accepting that I cannot control
my pain, I find that I no longer allow it to control me. I focus on
helping others whom I once viewed as weak, and help them to do
what they can to relinquish control of their pain as I am trying to
do. I stop thinking about trying to control my life or my pain —
instead I focus on being of service to others. By so doing,
I take the power away from my self-centered addiction and
self-absorbed pain. I gain a great reward.

*I relinquish control of my chronic pain by focusing on something
else: helping myself and others through pain recovery. In my
darkest moments, I become a light for others.*

CONCERN

PHYSICAL BALANCE

*"We are not so much concerned if you are slow
as when you come to a halt."*
Chinese proverb

Being "concerned" sounds so much more mature and
sophisticated than being worried, panicked, anxious, or scared,
but they all amount to much the same thing. However, I didn't
enter pain recovery to spend my time being "concerned," or any
of its synonyms, either—at least no more than absolutely necessary.

I work the steps of my pain recovery program to the best of my
ability today, and don't worry about results; I leave them to my
higher power. I follow the advice of my sponsor, counselor,
therapist, or others in recovery, and I expect results. I don't waste
time today being "concerned," or any other synonym for fear. I keep
moving through situations and issues in my life, sometimes slowly,
because that's the best I can do. But I keep working my program of
recovery. I don't stop. I just slow down sometimes.

*Concern today is something I show others—concern, consideration,
and caring. I have tools and a support group, and if I utilize them, I no
longer need to be concerned about my own serenity. That will come. It
may come slowly, but if I work my program, it will come.*

THINKING OF JOY

MENTAL BALANCE

....

*"As he slowed down and breathed, joy replaced anger
and anxiety; he relaxed and his pain diminished."*
A Day without Pain

Joy comes from being in balance. I go about my routines, focus
on exercise, reading, studying, and doing step work, or work
out of *Pain Recovery*. But when I focus my mind on things other
than quietly sitting, meditating, praying, or breathing, a couple of
days go by and I'm feeling restless. I'm not in touch with the joy
that is already inside me. It takes time, dedication, and focus of
the mind to listen to and feel that joy. If I'm not feeling it,
that's not because it's not there.

Joy is like my higher power—always there and waiting for me
to be open to that power. Joy is sitting patiently and waiting for me
to bring my thoughts to bear on it. There is joy for life, joy for living
without drugs, joy for my family and friends, even joy for my pain.
But when I'm not balanced mentally, I cannot feel the joy that is
in my heart. All other kinds of excitement, happiness, and freedom
with outside things and accomplishments are temporary. Joy is
permanent and never leaves me. It runs deep—as deep
as I'm willing to go to find it.

*I honor and acknowledge the joy I feel, even when I'm not feeling
it strongly. I take the time to make sure that my mind is in balance
and know that through my thoughts of a spiritual connection,
my joy is waiting for me.*

EMOTIONAL PAIN

EMOTIONAL BALANCE

"To regret one's own experiences is to arrest
one's own development. To deny one's own
experiences is to put a lie into the lips of one's life.
It is no less than a denial of the soul."

Oscar Wilde

Emotional pain can sometimes be as hurtful as the physical pain I have experienced as the result of my chronic pain condition. The emotional pain I've been through in active addiction while abusing pain medication became so great at times that I felt the need to use even more. The more emotional pain I experienced, the more out of emotional balance I was. I cannot achieve true, balanced recovery and live a life of meaning with chronic pain if I am not in balance. I experience pain as I go through life, just like everyone else. It is a natural part of living. Part of living life on life's terms is learning how to deal with and walk through not only physical pain, but emotional pain too. It helps to remember that, when I'm in emotional pain, this too shall pass.

*My emotional pain may be trying to teach me something;
it may be representing some unresolved issue I need to address
in my recovery program.*

TRIGGERS

SPIRITUAL BALANCE

....

"We should every night call ourselves to account:
What infirmity have I mastered today?
What passions opposed? What temptation resisted?
What virtue acquired?"
Seneca

Just about anything can trigger feelings in me today. Fear, anger, sadness, self-pity—any one of these painful emotions can be triggered by an innocent word, a song on the radio, a billboard I see as I drive to an appointment. I *could* respond the way I did before I entered pain recovery, and devote time and energy to "searching" within myself for the "cause" of the pain. (Somehow this never results in any new revelations, but it does keep me in pain as long as I continue to do it.) I can waste my mental energy trying to "heal a sick mind with a sick mind," as it's said in the rooms of recovery. Or I can do what my program tells me to do—I can search my soul for my own weaknesses, for the areas in which I may be dishonest, resentful, selfish, or fearful—in other words, spiritually unfit. And I can ask my higher power for forgiveness when I see my part in what is bothering me. I ask for forgiveness and I ask to have my attention directed to someone or something I can help.

Today I use triggers as a way to bring me closer to my higher power.
I focus on constant prayer, remembering the freedom I have today
from active addiction, and on positive thoughts that will
turn to positive action.

SECONDARY GAIN

RELATIONSHIPS

....

"Secondary gain refers to any perceived benefit
you receive from having pain. If not identified,
secondary gain gives you unconscious reasons
for holding onto your pain."
Pain Recovery: How to Find Balance and
Reduce Suffering from Chronic Pain

It took time for me to realize that I did receive a benefit from being
in chronic pain. Sometimes it was more than one benefit. I wasn't
"faking" my pain in order to receive these benefits…I wasn't even
aware I was receiving them until I entered recovery.

Some of these benefits included receiving more attention
from friends and family, being excused from having to work,
being relieved of responsibilities, getting out of unpleasant
activities, and having an excuse to take medication. I no longer
need to be in pain in order to receive benefits; in recovery today,
I can simply ask to have my legitimate needs met, being aware
of my expectations and wants in a healthy way, being productive
and working, taking responsibility, showing up for activities,
and not abusing medication.

I remember my responsibilities and expectations in my life.
I know that by not using my pain as an excuse to get the secondary
gain, I am actually reducing the intensity of the pain itself and
making it easier on myself. I find healthy ways to live through the
habits I create for myself to meet my expectations.

{ FEBRUARY }

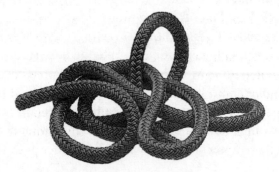

CONTROL

PHYSICAL BALANCE

....

"He who controls others may be powerful,
but he who has mastered himself is mightier still."
Tao Te Ching

Control. What a word. There was a time when I thought I
was in control, of myself and of the world and the people in it.
Paradoxically, that was during the time of my active addiction. Oh,
yes, I may have been "in control" of my emotions and my feelings,
but I was really just dulling them with medication so that I wouldn't
feel them. That was only the illusion of control, because ultimately,
my addiction had total control over me. It was my master.

Entering pain recovery, I was told I had to accept my powerlessness.
To me that sounded like admitting I couldn't be in control,
and I didn't like it. However, through abstaining from abuse of
medications, attending meetings, working steps with a sponsor, and
being of service to others, I began to see that the real way to regain
some kind of control over my life was to relinquish the need to
control my feelings by abusing medication. I began to feel a kind of
mastery over myself, ironically, when I gave up trying to control my
life or that of others. I leave that to my higher power today.

*I strive to keep my ego in check and make decisions based on my
actual, not perceived, needs as filtered through recovery, not through
my desires based on a distorted perspective of a self-image. I do not
allow my ego to control all aspects of my life today.*

LISTENING WITHIN

MENTAL BALANCE

*"Spend time every day listening
to what your muse is trying to tell you."*
St. Bartholomew

As I wake up in the morning, stretching my painfully stiff limbs, my mind starts to race. I hear others in the household or neighbors perhaps, getting ready for their days as I get up and get ready for mine. I know I dreamt last night, but the memories of my dreams are already slipping away as my head starts to clamor with plans for the day. Before I know it, I'm up and about and into my day, and I've forgotten to take the time to make contact with my higher power to ask for strength and guidance and hope.

Today, I must ask for help with my recovery, both from addiction and from my chronic pain. I must remember to ask for the help I need in the morning, if I want it throughout the day. And when the loving answer comes, I want it to find me listening.

*I take the time to focus my thoughts, to hear and listen to
the spirit inside me. That spirit is filled with joy, which today
I take time to notice and appreciate, whereas in the past I have
taken joy for granted. Joy comes when I focus my thoughts on
the body-mind-spirit connection.*

GRATITUDE

EMOTIONAL BALANCE

"Gratitude is not only the greatest of virtues,
but the parent of all the others."
Marcus Tullius Cicero

Not only has my pain negatively influenced all aspects of my
life, such as my thoughts, feelings, emotions, daily habits and
rituals, and even my connection to my higher power; it also has
detrimental effects on my attitude. Every day, I wake up and my
first thought is of my pain, wondering how it might influence
the rest of my day. I go to bed at night, again thinking of my pain,
and how it hindered me that day. Gratitude gets lost in the
midst of thoughts such as these.

Rather than dwelling on the negative, today I search for the
positive. I now wake up each day feeling blessed to be alive. My
pain reminds me each day that I am living, and from the moment
I realize that, I choose to live each day to the fullest, simply doing
the best I can. I take time to become more in tune with my spirit,
my thoughts, and my emotions. I embrace them each day for I
know I am alive and my higher power has a plan for me.

*Gratitude is everything. I know I cannot control the situations that
created my chronic pain, but I can control how I live each day. I take
control of my life and no longer let my pain control me. I am grateful
to be alive, even with my pain, just for right now.*

MOVEMENT TOWARD SPIRITUAL CONNECTION

SPIRITUAL BALANCE

*"I am not afraid of storms,
for I am learning how to sail my ship."*
Louisa May Alcott

In my active addiction, I had been in fear of making my pain worse, so I would make every attempt to move as little as possible. Early in my pain recovery, I was unaware of what would alleviate my pain and what would exacerbate it. Just thinking about getting out of bed or walking to the mailbox would cause my body to tense up in fear of the pain that was to come. While it's true that simple acts such as these may make my pain momentarily worse, going into them full of tension and fear only makes the pain that much more difficult to bear.

I have learned in recovery to work on improving my inner strength and my spiritual balance to help alleviate these fears. Movement is not my enemy, and I do not need to walk through my pain with any fear. I have a relationship with a higher power that takes each new step with me—physically, emotionally, mentally, and spiritually. Each day, each step, each new movement brings me new knowledge of the best ways to manage and live with my pain. As long as I am actively seeking this knowledge, I do not have any reason to fear movement.

I move about freely to the best of my ability. I embrace movement as my friend, and with each move I make in the physical world, I'm increasing my inner strength to handle a life with chronic pain.

SPIRITUAL PRINCIPLES

RELATIONSHIPS

....

"...becoming aware of the wishes, feelings,
and needs of others, and taking the needs
of others into consideration ..."
Adapted from Pain Recovery: How to Find Balance
and Reduce Suffering from Chronic Pain

A solution-oriented strategy to deal with my chronic pain is to develop a habit of thinking and acting that is consistent with the Serenity Prayer's guidance to "accept the things I cannot change," and that includes "the wishes, feelings, and needs of others."

Paradoxically, surrendering to the things I cannot control or change is necessary to reestablish the ability to choose how I want to act and what kind of life I want to have in recovery. One of the most important skills necessary to pain recovery is learning how to cope effectively with the often small, but irritating normal and natural frustrations of life.

*I am aware of the small, normal, frustrating aspects of life,
knowing that a spiritual awakening depends on my making a habit
of dealing with daily small struggles—including the wishes, feelings,
and needs of others—in ways that are consistent with the tools
and principles I'm learning in recovery.*

ACCEPTING FEELINGS

EMOTIONAL BALANCE

"Accepting your feelings takes less energy than trying to deny or suppress them. Also, accepting your feelings sometimes helps prevent them from recurring over and over and enables you to change them. Finally, fully accepting your feelings allows you to shift your energy to productive thoughts or actions."

Pain Recovery: How to Find Balance and Reduce Suffering from Chronic Pain

When I have emotional balance, I am free to feel my full emotional experience, recognizing that all my feelings are part of me. I don't avoid any of my feelings when I stay focused on being present in my body. I accept my emotions without labeling them good or bad, healthy or unhealthy.

Understanding that feelings are neither good nor bad (not judging my feelings), seeing that simply experiencing emotions does not hurt me, I know that feeling my emotions results in physical healing. By avoiding my feelings I know I will have ongoing suffering. Balanced thoughts and actions create balanced emotions.

Accepting my emotions, my feelings, frees me from my physical pain. My physical actions and habits lead to physical balance, which makes it possible for me to more fully feel the broad spectrum of my emotions; it's a loop. Through focus on physical habits I am acting in a way that allows me to be emotionally balanced.

JOY

MENTAL BALANCE

···

"Remember this—that very little
is needed to make a happy life."
Marcus Aurelius Antonius

Joy is a state of mind, and it comes in many ways. Sometimes it's just peace and contentment, serenity, inner connection to my higher power, and knowing that I'm in the right place. It's a smile or a laugh with friends and family. It's gratitude, knowing I'm in recovery today. It's the feeling I get when I finish working out or exercising. It's the warmth inside when I'm in a recovery meeting, listening to others share. It's a good meal, a good book, a film that moves me, a song that makes my heart sing along. But more than any of that, it's a state of mind. It's when my thoughts are directed at that which is fulfilling, uplifting, loving, and light in my life that joy floods in. It's just as important that I think joy as it is to feel joy. My physical pain may be minimal on any given day, but if my thoughts are directed at the negative, the darkness, then my body will surely go where my mind is already headed.

Pain doesn't have the power over me it once did. I've learned methods to cope with my pain that lessen its grip on me and my life. I use these methods to diminish my pain and increase my joy today.

GRIEF

EMOTIONAL BALANCE

....

"Waste not fresh tears on old griefs."
Alexander the Great

Grief can be frustrating, sad, draining, and painful. At times
it feels as though I don't even know myself when I'm in grief.
Pain recovery requires walking through all sorts of feelings, the
most severe of which is grief. I grieve the loss of my medications.
I grieve the loss of my pain as an excuse for my behavior. Being
in recovery, and in grief, I may not even recognize my behavior
as a reaction to feelings I may never have had to feel before,
when they were masked with drugs.

Grief over the loss of a person may be a little easier to identify
than grief over a lost behavior, place, or manner of being, but
each may be equally painful. Grief may be mixed with many other
feelings—anger, sadness, fear, self-pity…all of these feelings may
cycle and repeat until finally, I begin to feel forgiveness, and
that's when I think I can love again.

*I have learned that experiencing my feelings and accepting them has
allowed me to move through them. I don't need to waste "fresh tears on
old griefs." I feel my feelings and accept them as they are today.*

PRAYER AND MEDITATION

SPIRITUAL BALANCE

"And when ye stand praying, forgive, if ye have ought
against any: that your Father also which is in heaven
may forgive you your trespasses."

Jesus Christ

There are many kinds of prayer, and many kinds of meditation.
Both prayer and meditation are helpful, and both are needed:
The Eleventh Step says I need both, telling me to seek to improve
my conscious contact with my higher power by praying and
meditating. This is sometimes easier said than done. Perhaps when
my prayers seem ineffective it's because I'm not doing the things
I should in order to pray with the right spirit. This doesn't mean
I have to "get good" first, and then seek contact with my higher
power. But I must be in a place of love and tolerance of others
for my prayers to be most effective.

I don't approach my higher power asking for love and help
if I haven't shown the same to others in my life. Today I know
that prayer offered from a place of love and tolerance in my heart
is many times more effective than prayers offered from a place
of anger, selfishness, or fear.

*I pray for help with my recovery and for help in living with my pain.
I strive to treat others with love and respect, so my prayers can rise
from love, to love, with love.*

KINDNESS

RELATIONSHIPS

······

"Kindness in words creates confidence.
Kindness in thinking creates profundity.
Kindness in giving creates love."

Lao-Tzu

My pain has always had an impact on the lives of others, disrupting my life and the lives of those around me. In pain recovery I'm aware of that potential for disruption, and take responsibility for my pain. I get out of myself by acknowledging the impact of my pain upon others. I make a habit of showing kindness to others by striving to reduce the impact my pain has on them.

The quality of my relationships with others is important to me. I want them to be full of loving kindness, so that they will be characterized by confidence, profundity (depth), and love. Therefore I strive to make my words and actions kind, loving, and deep, knowing that the quality of my interactions with others depends on the way I treat them. If I'm not kind to others I will be alone with my addiction and my pain. I appreciate those who share my life with me and look for ways to help them.

I work to lessen the impact my pain has on others. I reduce my outward expressions of pain and help others by showing my appreciation for having them in my life.

FORGIVENESS

PHYSICAL BALANCE

*"Forgiveness is the fragrance the violet
sheds on the heel that has crushed it."*
Mark Twain

The quality of my forgiveness has a direct impact on my
physical balance. It is not just my forgiveness of others, but also
my forgiveness of myself. The more I hold onto resentment, anger,
or fear, the more it affects my own physical pain. My body holds
onto things, often when I'm not even conscious of doing so.
For this reason it's important to work the Twelve Steps to uncover,
discover, and recover those areas of my life that cause my pain,
grief, anger, and resentment toward myself and others. Forgiveness
is a process and not an event. It's not a destination at which I
arrive and all is well and forgotten. In reality, I may never forget,
and in fact, remembering can and does drive me to work harder,
to continue to work on my recovery. Remembering what has
happened gives me wisdom. Forgiving brings me relief
from my physical and emotional pain.

*I understand and have forgiveness for myself and others,
knowing that my level of forgiveness is related to the ability and
fortitude with which I work my program of recovery; and that affects
my health and level of pain.*

HONESTY

MENTAL BALANCE

....

"Honesty is the first chapter of the book of wisdom."
Thomas Jefferson

Honesty means more than simply telling the truth when prompted. Honesty means the acknowledgment of my chronic pain, addiction, and character defects. Honesty was perhaps the first spiritual principle I practiced when I admitted that maybe I had a problem with addiction. I practiced honesty when I looked at the unmanageability that abusing medication and acting on negative behaviors caused in my life and the lives of those I loved. Honesty is continuously required of me in my twelve-step work—otherwise the steps do not work.

Honesty, and my perception of its meaning, continues to evolve as I grow in pain recovery. The truth sets me free of my pain. In chronic pain and active addiction, those around me expected me to lie about how I was feeling to get what I needed. In recovery, those around me expect me to be honest about how I'm feeling and what I'm doing to get what I need.

I view honesty as a way to keep my mind, body, and spirit clear and free. I no longer view honesty as a duty, but an opportunity for growth. I welcome the expectation of honesty from those who support me in pain recovery.

COMMITMENT

EMOTIONAL BALANCE

....

*"Help me appreciate the rewards in my life
that flow from my commitments."*
Of Character: Building Assets in Recovery

There are days when my physical pain is small compared to the
emotional pain I experience when I contemplate that I might feel
physical pain for the rest of my life. Some days it seems the tears
will not stop, but only because I am caught in the trap of believing
that what I'm experiencing now is what I'll experience forever…
and forever seems like an unbearably long time.

Thinking this way keeps me mired in self-pity, which is simply
another manifestation of the selfishness I've learned is the root of
my problem. But how to get out of this self-pitying trap when my
physical and emotional pain seem to stretch in every direction
I can see? There is one way that never fails: helping or working
with others. I make a commitment to helping another person or
group. I agree to be a greeter at my home group or to read recovery
literature with a newcomer, and I keep my commitment. Soon
my "pity party" is over and I don't even realize how it happened.
Commitment is the key to service.

*Sometimes it's hard to think about a future without pain; thinking
about the future at all seems to bring thoughts that are hard to shake.
The solution I've found is to focus on helping another person today,
and I remain committed to my program of recovery.*

COURAGE
SPIRITUAL BALANCE

"Courage conquers all things;
it even gives strength to the body."
Roman proverb

Recovery takes courage. Disagreeing with my doctor and saying,
"No, I don't want any more pain medicine," or telling my still-using
friends I no longer want to hang out with them and get loaded
takes courage. All of these things require tremendous courage
on the part of a person in recovery.

It is during these difficult times that I ask my higher power
to give me the strength to do what needs be done for my recovery.
I draw strength from my family or others in recovery who have
walked the path before me; knowing that they can do it gives
me the courage I need to do it, too.

*I find the longer I am in recovery, the more I apply my program,
the deeper I discover a wealth of courage I never knew I had.
Recovery is simple, but not easy. My recovery fellowship, my sponsor,
and my higher power all give me the courage I need to work
my program every day.*

FORGIVENESS

EMOTIONAL BALANCE

"To hold on to resentments or grudges without forgiveness hurts only the one who holds them."
Recovery A to Z: A Handbook of
Twelve-Step Key Terms and Phrases

Sometimes it's hard to accept my chronic pain. Sometimes I actually blame myself for my pain; I need to forgive myself for feeling the pain I sometimes feel.

It's as if, in my dreams, I envisioned having a child who would play ball, run, and climb, but instead I have one who cannot do such things. Would I judge such a child harshly for what he or she couldn't do, or would I celebrate and praise him or her for the things that he or she could accomplish? Part of physical forgiveness is finding, creating, and maintaining habits that are within the bounds of what my body *can* do, and doing those things as a way to show forgiveness toward myself. If the things I can do today are not the things I was able to do in the past, so be it. I forgive myself for my disabilities today, and celebrate my abilities with gratitude.

I love myself enough today, the way I would a small child. I forgive my broken body and ask it to forgive me for all the times I haven't taken care of it as well as I could have. Today, I do what I can, and I am grateful. I take care of my body today, as I would a small child.

GRIEF

PHYSICAL BALANCE

....

"The cure for grief is motion."
Elbert Hubbard

Grief can happen weeks, months, even years after I experience a loss. It can even come, seemingly, when I am in the middle of doing everything I need to be doing for my recovery. It may come out of nowhere and strike so suddenly that I don't have time to put up a defense against it. I can stand still and wonder what happened, getting lost in the feeling, or I can keep walking forward, literally as well as figuratively, making myself move, exercise, and walk, putting one foot in front of the other, in my program of recovery and in my physical life as well. I do this and trust that over time, through action, therapy, sponsorship, meeting attendance, and writing/working steps, as well as through prayer and meditation, the feelings of grief will be lifted, as long as I continue to work my program of recovery.

I handle my feelings of grief today, even when I'm not sure of their cause, by focusing on the four points of balance. I don't let my feelings of grief affect my physical balance—I do what needs to be done so I can reveal, discover, and heal.

SERENITY

PHYSICAL BALANCE

"Maintaining balance in your physical life entails
continuous monitoring, but not judgment, about your
state of nutrition, energy, exercise patterns,
and ingestion of toxins. Maintaining physical balance
involves monitoring your body as well as emotions
associated with your body."
Adapted from Pain Recovery: How to Find Balance
and Reduce Suffering from Chronic Pain

Serenity is directly connected to my physical body and my habits.
I make a habit of taking care of my body by doing yoga, stretching,
going for a walk, or exercising in ways that work for me, based on
the help and counsel of my physical therapist or a doctor who is
familiar with my physical condition. If I'm not feeling particularly
serene in pain recovery, chances are I'm neglecting some of my
healthy physical habits—I'm not taking care of myself. When this
happens, my serenity is usually the first thing to go, followed quickly
by my temper. But I can retrieve my serenity through working
my program and reinforcing my healthy habits.

*My level of serenity is directly connected to the physical habits
I maintain today. Serenity itself is a healthy habit that requires
I maintain my spiritual fitness.*

CONTROL
EMOTIONAL BALANCE

....

"Be not angry that you cannot make others
as you wish them to be, since you cannot
make yourself as you wish to be."
Thomas à Kempis

Think of a handful of sand—the harder I try to hold on to it,
and the more I squeeze, the faster the grains run through my
fingers. Trying to exert control over people and events in my
life is like trying to hold onto a handful of sand; the more I
squeeze, the less I end up with.

I have control over what I say and do; pretty much everything else
in the world is out of my control. I may influence people with
words and actions, but I don't have control over them.

I can make plans, but I can't control the results. I do "the footwork"
and leave the results up to my higher power. The knowledge that
I am not in control is actually a great relief. When I stop believing
I control the outcomes of my efforts, and just try to do the next
right thing, my emotional state becomes more relaxed. Knowing
I'm responsible only for my actions, and not for the results of my
actions, is a source of emotional balance in my recovery.

*It is important to be loving and good to myself by taking an honest look
at what I have control over and surrendering what I don't.*

LACK OF TRUST

SPIRITUAL BALANCE

"You may be deceived if you trust too much,
but you will live in torment unless you trust enough."
Frank Crane

Trust is an experience. It may be the experience of sharing intimate details of my life with another. It may be the experience of keeping another's confidence after they have shared with me.

Trust is built by taking right actions, repeatedly, sometimes even when I don't quite see how doing so will help me with either my pain or my addiction. However, I see others in recovery taking these same actions and recovering; so I trust that these actions will work for me.

When I lack trust, taking right action seems almost impossible. I ask my higher power to help me trust that I can recover, that I can walk through my pain without abusing medications. I replace lack of trust with trust, by taking right actions and experiencing the results.

I understand trust is more than a feeling; it is the action I take of opening up and sharing with another person, listening to and following another's suggestion, and continuing to stay in the pain recovery process.

CONCERN
RELATIONSHIPS

....

"The ability to give back is a gift that recovery provides.
When you get out of yourself, it helps you to see your
problems in the proper perspective and context."

Pain Recovery: How to Find Balance and
Reduce Suffering from Chronic Pain

Am I making a habit of demonstrating concern or caring for others
when I am at a recovery group meeting, or am I always making
everything about me? Am I sharing to talk about my own pain to
get attention, or to help others find a solution?

I can start showing concern for others from the very beginning of
my recovery. If I'm not picking up the telephone because I don't
want to talk to anyone, why don't I make it a habit to pick up the
phone to listen? Soon, I can make it a habit to call others to see
how they are doing. I ask others how they are progressing in their
pain recovery program. At first I may do this to create an opening so
I can talk about myself. But soon, I find myself genuinely showing
others the concern that I want people to show for me. I listen, not
providing advice or direction, but just to lend an ear that others
can talk to. I know the isolation that comes from chronic pain and
active addiction. I know the loneliness of early recovery. I can show
concern for others on that same path by extending myself to others
who are in the process of recovery as well.

I make a habit of demonstrating concern for the welfare of others. Part
of my daily routine is to get out of myself and show, by my actions, I
care for another who is recovering from chronic pain and addiction.

PATIENCE

PHYSICAL BALANCE

"Patience is the companion of wisdom."
St. Augustine

When I'm in pain, I want it to stop. Right now. Pain medications might give me that immediate relief I crave; however, the damage they may do to my recovery means they are no longer an option for me. I have to use the tools of pain recovery today in order to take care of my disease of addiction as well as my pain. And that takes a lot of patience.

Because today I seek relief in the principles embodied in the Twelve Steps rather than in pain medication, I must be patient. I've learned that twelve-step recovery works if I work it; however, it is not as quick as a pill. If I expect immediate results from my efforts to reduce or eliminate my pain, my expectations may lead to frustration and disappointment, because practicing twelve-step principles, though ultimately effective, takes longer than pain medications. This is why patience is so important.

Impatient expectations only cause my pain to get worse. My worsening pain then tests my patience. The vicious cycle of pain and impatience spins to increase physical and emotional suffering. When I am able to muster even the smallest amount of acceptance and display the least bit of patience, I soon discover that my pain lessens.

I use the tools available to learn patience and reduce my stress and pain. I learn from others in the program how to develop necessary coping skills. Patience brings progress. As long as I take a step in the right direction and do it slowly, patience finds me.

GRATITUDE

MENTAL BALANCE

....

"Now that I'm in recovery I don't fantasize about dying
or dread the thought of living. I wake up each day
grateful for another twenty-four hours clean and look
forward toward the unfolding day with anticipation."
Tails of Recovery: Addicts and the Pets That Love Them

Waking up each day with gratitude does not mean that I don't
wake some mornings with some anxiety or a little stress about the
day ahead. What it means to wake up with gratitude for me is that
I take the time to remember what I'm glad to have in my life —
recovery, family, friends, a program. How different from when
I was in active addiction, before I entered recovery. Then, I would
wake up and think of all the difficult things that lay ahead of me:
this doctor appointment, that lab test, my pain and how
I'm going to suffer through the day.

Today, I bring to mind the good things in my life, and I get to
the other stuff later. First-things-first today means focusing on the
gratitude in my life. That attitude carries me through my day,
regardless of how I'm feeling or what kind of day is ahead of me.

*Gratitude is a state of mind more than anything else. I keep gratitude
in my mind and think of things that I am grateful for, whether I am
feeling grateful or not; I still know I have much to be grateful for.*

ALL FEELINGS ARE TEMPORARY

EMOTIONAL BALANCE

"Sometimes I think I shouldn't feel the way I do. When I start thinking this way I tell myself that feelings are neither good nor bad—they simply are. In the midst of intense negative feelings, whether fear, anger, depression, etc., it can feel as though they will last forever, like they will never end. It promotes emotional balance to maintain an awareness that all feelings are temporary, and that they always change."

Adapted from Pain Recovery: How to Find Balance and Reduce Suffering from Chronic Pain

Emotional balance is achieved when I allow myself to feel whatever comes up, and learn to accept my feelings without judging them. Because my feelings are a part of me, accepting them as they are is an important part of accepting myself as I am. This is also known as self-acceptance. Whatever positive change I want to make in my life, acceptance of how and where I am at in the present moment is one of the keys to moving forward. Accepting my feelings also takes less energy than trying to avoid or suppress them, and helps me maintain balance by eliminating the need for them to persist. Genuine acceptance of my feelings gives me the opportunity to shift my energy to thoughts and actions that facilitate the learning, growing, and healing that can fuel the continuing progress of my pain recovery.

I have learned to practice strategies to identify and express emotions in ways that promote balance; deal with distressing, uncomfortable feelings in healthy ways; and strengthen positive feelings to promote growing, healing, and recovery.

LOVING KINDNESS

SPIRITUAL BALANCE

"The highest wisdom is loving kindness."
The Talmud

I once used the word "concern" to describe how I felt about my pain and my body's well-being. However, a dictionary defines concern as "anxiety, worry, apprehension, fear, alarm, distress, or unease." So concern is really another level of fear, and today, I don't want to live in fear, of my pain or anything else. So I am not concerned about my body today; I show it loving kindness instead.

When I begin to be concerned for my pain level, I reach into my tools of pain recovery and I remember to feel gratitude for having a higher power in my life. I reach out to help others, thus enlarging my spiritual life and connectedness, especially when the physical, mental, and emotional pain is more than I believe I can handle.

When my pain seems overwhelming, I don't become concerned.
Instead, I act out of loving kindness for myself and focus outward,
on what I can do for others; knowing that I can manage my pain,
I can live with the feeling, and if I get through today,
tomorrow can and will be better.

COMMITMENT

RELATIONSHIPS

....

"This is the mark of a really admirable man:
steadfastness in the face of trouble."
Ludwig van Beethoven

Commitment means many things to many people.
Commitments can be big, such as getting married or joining
the military. Commitment can also mean agreeing to make coffee
at a meeting or to serve as a greeter at the door. Commitment,
whether big or small, is very important—it's an opportunity
for me to be of service to others.

Commitment allows me to get up, suit up, and show up. These
necessary steps allow me to stay in contact with my support network
and to continue with my pain recovery.

I view commitment as a positive step toward pain recovery.
I make commitments consistent with my availability and ability,
but I do make commitments. Commitment means being there
for others, because they were there for me. Paying forward to
pay back is my new commitment.

I volunteer for a service commitment when I see the need.
The commitment can be simple and for a short duration, but
I make a commitment to a twelve-step group or meeting.

SANITY

MENTAL BALANCE

"Order is the sanity of the mind, the health of the body,
the peace of the city, the security of the state. Like beams
in a house or bones to a body, so is order to all things."
Robert Southey

Sanity today means dealing with pain without using addictive drugs;
I deal sanely, that is to say, in an orderly way, with my pain.

Before I entered recovery, I lived in the disorder and insanity of
using addictive pain medication. Drug addiction was both a result
of and a way to cope with my chronic pain. The drugs worked for
a short time, or so I thought, as I spiraled into disorder and out
of control. Then came the insanity—I thought more drugs were
the answer. Now I understand that the drugs only compounded
my problem. Through the help of my support group and an
understanding counselor, therapist, sponsor, and program friends,
I continue my journey into recovery. The Twelve Steps, recovery-
oriented literature, and others who share in my life are sources of
sanity. As long as I continue to make progress by focusing on my
physical, mental, emotional, and spiritual balance, and on keeping
my life balanced and in order, my concept and understanding
of sanity become clearer.

*I work my program, focusing on balance, so I can continue
to learn and grow. Mental balance restores me to sanity—when
and if I follow my healthy routines and listen to the advice of
others in recovery who guide me.*

FLEXIBILITY

MENTAL BALANCE

....

*"We challenge you to give up
what is not helping you with your pain."*
A Day without Pain

When I'm in pain it's usually a result of holding onto something long after the "expiration date." I'm learning that being flexible enough to risk letting go—of fears, resentments, and expectations—is necessary if I'm to shift from pain to freedom.

I practice flexibility in a variety of ways, like doing something I wouldn't normally do—maybe I drive home a different way one day, or listen to a different radio station in the car. I listen to someone like my sponsor, therapist, counselor, or others in my pain recovery program, and allow their suggestions into my life. I step gently outside my comfort zone, to the very edge of my capability (but never over it into increased pain). Flexibility is an exercise of my mind. I practice going with the flow and accepting what's coming or going in my life, rather than holding on and trying to control things in order to get what I want. Through practicing flexibility, I'm opening up to and living in the possibility that my emotional pain does not last forever and my chronic pain does not rule my life.

I'm flexible with my plans and ideas about my life and what is good for me. When an idea's time has passed, I'm flexible enough to let go and move on. Where I would normally say "no," today I may practice saying "yes," and where I may normally say "yes," I may say "no." I'll do something that someone with experience in pain recovery suggests, regardless of my personal, comfort-based objections.

CULTIVATING POSITIVE STATES OF MIND

EMOTIONAL BALANCE

....

*"It is our attitude at the beginning of
a difficult task which, more than anything else,
will affect its successful outcome."*

William James

I work on creating positive states of mind today in order to improve my attitude. One way I do this is by remembering to be grateful for my life today. And a great way to cultivate an attitude of gratitude is by writing a list of the four or five things I'm most grateful for each night before I go to sleep. And because I take this action to cultivate a positive state of mind, today I have a degree of emotional balance that helps me as I perform the tasks of recovery: prayer, meditation, meeting attendance, working the steps, and service.

Sometimes I look at a gratitude list from a month or a year ago and see what things have changed. My gratitude lists help me maintain a positive attitude by showing me that I do have much to be grateful for. As long as I work my program of recovery, my attitude of gratitude will help me cultivate and maintain the positive state of mind so necessary for my recovery.

I cultivate, honor, and nurture a positive state of mind, knowing that when my attitude and mind-set are strong and positive I have a better chance of living peacefully with my chronic pain.

SEPARATING PAIN
FROM SUFFERING
SPIRITUAL BALANCE

"Man suffers most from the suffering he fears, but
(which) never appears, therefore he suffers more
than God meant him to suffer."
Dutch proverb

My pain manifests itself in many forms—physical, emotional,
mental, and spiritual. Today I know the difference between pain
and suffering. Chronic pain is part of my physical life, while
emotional, mental, and spiritual pain can become suffering
if I allow myself to dwell in them.

Emotional, mental, and spiritual pains are real, just as real as the
chronic pain I feel in my body. I can take positive actions to lessen
or rid myself of chronic physical pain, but if I wallow or dwell in my
emotional, mental, and spiritual pain, then suffering is the result.

How to handle my suffering? The same way I handle my chronic
physical pain: healthy habits and reaching out to others—including
my higher power, my sponsor, my counselor, my fellowship. I
alleviate my suffering with balance in my life; I don't become too
focused on myself. I keep a healthy balance between self
and others, and my suffering diminishes.

*For today, just today, I see my pain for what it is and I see
my emotions for what they are. I strive to separate the two
and to deal with each separately.*

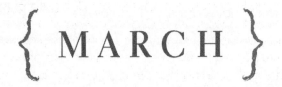

{ MARCH }

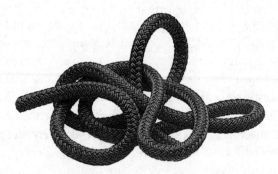

LOVE

RELATIONSHIPS

....

"Love, when truly felt and practiced, seldom brings our
needs in conflict with the needs of our loved ones. In
love, the importance of mutual needs is greater than
individual needs. On the rare occasion when mutual
and individual needs conflict, being loving requires
that we put our loved one's interests ahead of our own.
In doing so, we find that our mutual good is far more
important and fulfilling than our individual desires."

Of Character: Building Assets in Recovery

Love is my quest for the best and highest good. The idea of putting
another person's needs ahead of my own may sound codependent.
However, what I find during this surrender is that what I was
holding onto and perceiving as my own need was not real. In
surrendering to the need of another person I discover that acting
on the spiritual principles of love and kindness does not put me
in conflict with myself. I believe that the best and highest good
for another person cannot possibly be harmful to me. My task in
recovery is to discover that best and highest good. When there is
conflict, there is a lack of understanding of what that good is.

*Love is my quest, and seeking through prayer, meditation,
and communication to discover, to reveal, and to act in the best
and highest good for myself and others, transcending all conflict
of needs, both real and perceived.*

SELF-CARE

PHYSICAL BALANCE

....

"Well-ordered self-love is right and natural."
Thomas Aquinas

"If one is good, two must be better." That's the way I thought in active addiction. Today I know that too much of even a good thing isn't always good for me. The book *Pain Recovery* taught me that. For example, embarking on a too-vigorous course of exercise that might result in injury; losing weight by starving myself; engaging in myriad activities that I haven't tried before, such as acupuncture, massage, physical therapy, or chiropractic, without a developing a consistent plan; or spending money and time on treatments and medications in excess of what's recommended or right for me are examples of the kinds of behavior I engaged in during my active addiction and from which I am now in recovery. I want to recover—now! So shouldn't I do everything possible to make that happen, now?

Maybe not, or at least not all at once. Caring for myself and showing myself healthy self-love means taking things easy and letting my higher power do those things for me that I cannot do for myself. I follow the steps of my program, and do what is necessary for good health. I eat healthy foods, sleep and rest when I can, and I get some exercise. I also work my program of recovery, praying and meditating and being of service, and letting my higher power do the rest.

Taking care of myself today means doing what I see others in pain recovery doing successfully: eating, sleeping, exercising, praying, and meditating. I ask my higher power to help me with the rest, and I have faith that my request will be answered.

COURAGE

MENTAL BALANCE

....

*"Courage is resistance to fear, mastery of fear—
not absence of fear."*
Mark Twain

In the Serenity Prayer I ask for courage. But what does courage really mean? It's not the absence of fear; I've learned that. Courage in pain recovery, as in all of life, is doing the right thing in spite of fear. I apply courage in all four points of balance. In relation to my thoughts, mental courage is twofold: it is the courage to ignore negative thinking, and it is the ability to think of something new and different, or in a new way.

I practice courage on a mental level by replacing negative, "what's the use" thoughts with the affirmations, thoughts, and ideas of recovery. I practice having positive thoughts. I practice thinking healthy thoughts. I practice replacing negative ideas with positive ones, and then I put those ideas into action by doing what must be done regardless of what I think, what I fear, how I feel.

This is what it means to have courage, and this is how I change the things that I can. I can change what I do. I can change what I think. In changing what I think and what I do, I can change the way I feel.

*I might not ever be able to remove my chronic pain, but
I can change my thinking about my pain. In changing my thinking,
I change my actions. I practice courage in all points of balance
and I dare to think differently.*

SELF-PITY

EMOTIONAL BALANCE

"Self-pity is defined as excessive, self-absorbed unhappiness over one's own troubles. It is the emotional state of feeling sorry for myself, sometimes in exaggerated ways. Self-pity is often a characteristic of chronic pain and addiction—after all, these troubles are very real. But the fact that self-pity often results from significant problems does not make it any less destructive in terms of its impact on emotional balance. When I'm feeling self-pity, I'm almost exclusively focused on what is wrong and not working in my life."

Adapted from Pain Recovery: How to Find Balance
and Reduce Suffering from Chronic Pain

A solution-oriented way to regain emotional balance when I'm feeling sorry for myself is to make a gratitude list. This can help me regain perspective and disrupt excessive focus on the negative. I can identify things in my life that I'm grateful for. This does not need to discount the areas of my life that I want to improve or that I'm working on. This does not mean that it's not okay to have problems or still wish for things to be better. After all, I continue on the path of recovery because I want continued improvement in my life. But ironically, that improvement comes through being grateful for what I do have today.

I am grateful for what I have today, even if that is just the willingness to improve the areas of my life that may still need some time and attention. I am grateful for where I've come from, where I am today, and where I'm going.

TRUST

RELATIONSHIPS

....

"As we do the things required of us to recover, we
begin to trust the people who help us, the program,
and our higher power. This often provides us with the
reassurance we need to trust the world."
Of Character: Building Assets in Recovery

In early recovery, I heard about the need to trust my higher
power, but I was definitely not used to trusting anyone. But I had
enough desperation to try. I was hoping to find someone I could
trust, who would keep private whatever I shared with him or her.
But I didn't discover that person until I took a little risk
and changed my old ways in order to find out.

I was desperate enough to try to trust, but as the desperation of early
recovery wears off, so the willingness to trust can decrease. That's
why it's so fortunate that I began to trust early on. By the time I had
a little recovery under my belt, I had begun building a little bit of
trust in the process. Today I know how and whom to trust.

I get to remember those times of desperation as reassurance when I'm
embarking on another level of trust in recovery. I start with recovery
and learn to trust myself. In trusting myself, I trust the world.

At any and all stages of recovery, I take the action first and develop trust
over time. In trusting one person in recovery who guides me and provides
suggestions, I develop trust in a higher power. Trusting a higher power
helps me trust myself. In trusting myself, I learn to trust others.

EXERCISE, MOVEMENT

PHYSICAL BALANCE

....

"The less we move, the more pain we have when
we do move, causing us to move less. It becomes
a vicious and painful cycle. The only solution for this
'un-movement syndrome' is moving."
Adapted from A Day without Pain

When I'm in pain, I feel inclined to rest and avoid exercise; however, exercise is one of the best things I can do to reduce my pain, as I learned in the book *Pain Recovery*. The danger of inactivity is that my body becomes de-conditioned, which can add substantially to my perception and experience of pain. Studies have shown that regular and sustained physical activity is beneficial to virtually every system in my body. During exercise, my body releases chemicals called endorphins, which naturally relieve pain and also help to lessen my anxiety and depression. The four major types of exercise are cardiovascular, strength training, balance, and stretching.

Other benefits of regular exercise are that it helps me to maintain a healthy weight, increases my flexibility so I don't strain muscles and joints, helps me build strength, increases my serotonin levels, which improves my mood and fights my pain, and protects and strengthens my heart and circulatory system while increasing my dopamine levels, which results in improving my mood and giving me energy.

I make sure to exercise because not only is it good for my recovery today, it is insurance for tomorrow.

CONTROL

MENTAL BALANCE

....

"These seemingly natural, automatic thoughts…
'self-talk'…define(s) your beliefs…While you may be
powerless over the self-talk that first enters your mind, you
are not powerless over what you do in response to it."

Pain Recovery: How to Find Balance and
Reduce Suffering from Chronic Pain

I take the action I need to take in my recovery, and sometimes
that means choosing to intervene on negative thoughts. I have
control over the continuing thought process that leads to physical,
emotional, and spiritual imbalance. Through working the steps
with a sponsor, therapist, or counselor, I become aware of the
slippery slope of thoughts that eventually leads to actions that
increase my pain, be it physical or emotional.

Certain thoughts lead directly to active addiction. I'm not
responsible and have no control over the first thought, but I have
the power to intervene on that thought and replace it with thoughts
of recovery. I've learned to take appropriate action and continue to
learn positive affirmations to replace negative thinking. When
I'm thinking of ways to control situations, people, or my chronic
pain, I surrender by stopping the thought-stream and replacing
it with recovery-minded thinking.

*I have control over how long I think something. I'm not responsible
for the first thought, but I'm responsible for what follows. I replace
negative thinking with positive affirmations. I have control over that
which I choose to affirm in my life today.*

TOXIC FEELINGS

EMOTIONAL BALANCE

....

"I count him lost who is lost to shame."
Plautus

In the book *Pain Recovery*, I discovered ways to deal with toxic feelings like shame and guilt. Just because I work a program of recovery, I'm not immune to either of these toxic feelings.

I know I'm feeling shame or guilt when I
catch myself in thoughts like these:

- I should be more patient with my spouse and kids; it's not their fault that I'm in pain.
- I should be back at work by now.
- I shouldn't be in this much pain.
- What's wrong with me?

When I'm dealing with shame and guilt (either giving it or getting it), I need to stop and review the tools I already have. I start by describing my own strengths and positive qualities. I identify any lies that other people have told me about myself that I can stop believing. Then I can discover (and remember) how to use this information to maintain better emotional balance. Whether I'm shaming others or feeling shame, I remember what I've learned, and change my feelings by thinking positively.

I'm in recovery, and don't need to feel shame for who I am. My pain recovery program teaches me that I can live differently today; that I no longer have to do things I later feel shame over; that I can make positive choices today that make me feel good inside.

MARCH

9

PURPOSE IN LIFE
SPIRITUAL BALANCE

"Life without a purpose is a languid, drifting thing;
every day we ought to review our purpose, saying to
ourselves, 'This day let me make a sound beginning,
for what we have hitherto done is naught!'"
Thomas à Kempis

Before my chronic pain struck, I felt like I had some purpose in my life. My family, work, school, sports, activities, etc., all gave meaning to my life. However, in my pain, my purpose became just getting through another day or moment.

My purpose seemed to become an effort to get everyone around me to understand just what I was feeling, even if I had to lash out and get others to actually feel pain along with me.

The physical pain spiraled into the mental, the mental into the emotional, and ultimately, a crisis of faith and spiritual connection ensued. But in pain recovery, I have purpose again after all this time, and it is not just to get through another day with pain. Instead, my purpose is to live my recovery, share my experience, and help another find and fulfill his or her purpose.

The foundation and fabric of the Twelve Steps is service and carrying a message, helping another. Getting out of myself was really what I sought through the abuse of medication; I've found another way to do that by helping others.

I have a purpose in life—staying in pain recovery and helping others. Everything else is built upon that.

CARING

RELATIONSHIPS

"...the essence of nursing is to help a patient, whether ill or well, live as independently as possible by helping him perform the daily activities he would otherwise perform if he had the necessary strength and ability."

Of Character: Building Assets in Recovery

It's natural and instinctive for some people to take care of themselves—not me. As a result of active addiction, I lost the ability to care for myself in healthy, loving, humane ways. I lost the instinct to provide for my needs. Things as simple as eating, grooming, resting, and recreation—normal human experiences—became secondary to fixing my chronic pain with the abuse of pain medication.

As a result of recovery, I make an effort to care for myself, making conscious, concerted efforts to do things for myself. Part of self-care is being disciplined with the care I provide, going out of my way to make sure to monitor that I'm caring for myself, until doing so becomes second nature again. Eventually the brain will rewire, and doing things for myself will once again become habitual. Until that time, my physical health is too important for me to ignore the discipline of caring for myself.

I provide myself with the care my body deserves, until my body can care for itself, so that I can do the right things for myself as a matter of course.

LOSS OF FUNCTION/ REGAINING FUNCTION

PHYSICAL BALANCE

"'Tis a lesson you should heed, Try, try again. If at first you don't succeed, Try, try again."
T. H. Palmer

Every day I'm in recovery I strengthen my ability to live with my pain, and as a result, I strengthen my ability to function. Whereas in the beginning of my recovery there were things I could not even dream of doing, today I can do some of those things with ease. For example, it used to be next to impossible for me to complete doing the laundry. As I progressed in recovery, I was able to get it started but not able to finish it in the same day. Today I can work on starting *and* finishing this simple-but-somehow-difficult household task, and when I master it, I can add others. I can work on increasing my own functioning. Maybe today will be the day I go for a walk with some of my work colleagues at lunchtime, rather than staying in my office because I think I'm in too much pain to go for that walk. Even if I don't succeed in regaining complete functioning today, I will know I tried.

I will choose something to do today that is outside my level of comfort, something I could not do in active addiction, and seek to complete that task. Through actions like this, I work on increasing my function, bit by bit.

CONCERN
MENTAL BALANCE

"If you believe that feeling bad or worrying long enough
will change a past or future event, then you are residing
on another planet with a different reality system."
William James

Concern can be a form of fear or worry—we say things like
"I'm concerned about your grades," or "I'm concerned about
traveling so late at night," meaning we have fears or negative
feelings about these things. But concern can be positive, too.
I have concern for the feelings or well-being of others today.

Being concerned about myself or others can be negative or
positive, productive or counterproductive. I become negatively
concerned about those things I have no real control over, but that
I obsess about anyway, giving myself the illusion I am doing
something about a problem or situation—this provides a handy, but
ultimately useless, distraction from the here and now. I need to think,
"What am I avoiding by wasting time on these fears?" I try to
have faith instead of fear.

Positive concerns are those things I do have the immediate ability
to do something about, mostly my own well-being: physical,
mental, emotional, and spiritual.

*I focus on positive concerns and leave the negative concerns for another
day. I let my higher power have control over those negative concerns
and ask that higher power for the courage, power, and strength to
help me with my positive concerns.*

NOT GUILTY
EMOTIONAL BALANCE

....

"Having chronic pain reinforces my shame and
can in and of itself become shame-inducing along
the lines of, I have this problem so there's obviously
something wrong with me.... Shame is self-defeating
to the point of being self-destructive."

Adapted from Pain Recovery: How to Find Balance
and Reduce Suffering from Chronic Pain

Guilt is emotional distress or discomfort based on the belief that there is a problem related to my behavior. Shame is the distress I feel when I believe there is something wrong, not with my behavior, but with me. Shame and guilt have their places—they can help me regulate my behavior with the intent of conforming to my own values or a more universal moral code. However, false or toxic guilt is a sense of responsibility for mistakes or problems for which I am not responsible. Feelings of toxic shame and guilt serve no useful purpose—in fact, they may be manifestations of a grandiose ego: "Look how 'bad' I am, I'm responsible for *everything!*" No, I don't need shame and guilt in my recovery—in fact, today I plead "not guilty" to things I'm not actually guilty of—however, I do take responsibility for my own actions.

I will feel less shame and guilt as I progress in recovery, working through the steps with a sponsor, and making amends for those wrongs for which I am actually responsible; then I will not have to carry shame or guilt for imagined wrongs in which I have no real part.

*I don't need to be ashamed of or guilty about my pain or my addiction
now that I am working a program of recovery.*

MONITORING AND WARNING SIGNS

SPIRITUAL BALANCE

"With spiritual balance…you are able to deal with
whatever life brings you and know you are okay.
You are able to find meaning and purpose even in
situations that are painful and not to your liking."
Adapted from Pain Recovery: How to Find Balance
and Reduce Suffering from Chronic Pain

Signs of spiritual balance include having a sense of purpose in life, being
able to trust, having faith, having feelings of connectedness to others and
to God/Spirit/my higher power. It is not likely early in my recovery that I
will immediately experience all of these feelings all the time, but slowly
but surely they will come, and, wonder of wonders, they will persist for
longer and longer periods of time the longer I stay in recovery.

Everyone feels lost, adrift, or isolated at times—these feelings are
part of being human. I don't have to worry about being in spiritual
imbalance if I experience these feelings at times—it's when they
persist to the point that they prevent me from getting back into
spiritual balance that a problem arises.

I can live in spiritual imbalance as long as I choose to, or
I can do the things that I know will get me back into spiritual balance:
prayer, meditation, reading recovery or other spiritual literature,
and being of service.

*I monitor myself for signs of spiritual imbalance without becoming
obsessed with restoring it. When I get stuck in spiritual imbalance,
I get out of myself by working with a sponsor or helping another,
whether that person is in my recovery program or not.*

COMMITMENT

RELATIONSHIPS

....

"As we grow and work the Twelve Steps, we develop
meaningful commitments to ourselves, others, and the
world...being committed to someone else, something
else, or ourselves requires much of us. It requires
we accept uncertainty in our lives, as well as the
uncertainty of who our friend or lover will become as
he or she grows and changes in ways unknown to us."
Of Character: Building Assets in Recovery

I'm not the only one who has changed as a result of being in
recovery and working the Twelve Steps. It seems everyone around
me has also changed as a result. Even though the changes due to
recovery are ultimately positive, all change is difficult. Even the
people who desperately wanted me to change now don't know how
to deal with "the new me" at times. That's okay. It takes us all some
time to adjust to leaving behind what had become comfortable,
even if it was unproductive or dangerous—at least it was familiar.

My commitment to my recovery is that I stay the course, even
when it seems like I'm way too far outside my comfort zone—
or that of others in my life.

*I'm committed to myself, my health, my recovery, regardless of what
anyone around me thinks, does, or says to try to discourage me. I
stick with my sponsor, my program, my counselors, and my recovery
fellowship; ultimately those who have my best interests at heart will
come to understand. Even if they don't, I'm committed to my recovery.*

MONITORING DRUG USE

PHYSICAL BALANCE

"Use, do not abuse..."
Voltaire

Not all medications are bad for me today, as the book *Pain Recovery* points out. When I'm taking any necessary medications, I ask myself what effect I'm expecting and experiencing. Taking an extra vitamin for energy or a muscle relaxant to decrease anxiety is not addiction, but might underlie a thinking style that looks for a psychological effect or relief from a drug. Many medications are not habit-forming and may be prescribed as part of a pain management plan; these include muscle relaxants, antiseizure medicines, and antidepressants. If they are prescribed, I take them with care and under the supervision of a health professional who is knowledgeable about recovery and chronic pain, and with the knowledge and advice of my sponsor.

It is important for me to remain mindful of the effects of any medications I'm taking, as well as their possible interactions with other prescription and over-the-counter medications. On a regular basis, I make a list of the medications that I'm using, and I discuss them with my support group. I never have the luxury of being casual about my potential to relapse. My recovery requires constant vigilance.

I take a look at any and all drugs or supplements I'm taking, including vitamins and over-the-counter drugs, and ask myself why I'm taking them, if I really need to be taking them, or if I could get the same benefit from behavioral changes instead. I discuss these questions with my counselor, therapist, sponsor, or someone else in pain recovery.

ACTIONS
MENTAL BALANCE

"The actions of men are
the best interpreters of their thoughts."
John Locke

I cannot think my way into a better way of living. I have to live my way into a better way of thinking. I may not think positive thoughts about my pain today, but over time those thoughts change. I start the process of recovery through action. After acting a certain way I start to feel better and my thought process begins to change.

Regardless of how I think on any given day, the actions that I take are what matters. I may think that I'm not getting better. I may think this process does not seem to be working. I may even think it's pointless to exercise, meditate, or go to a recovery group today. Learning how to not listen to my thoughts and to take positive, appropriate action instead is key to pain recovery.

I take the appropriate action for where I am in my recovery today. I do not listen to my negative thoughts. I know that if I take the right action, my thought process will change.

SHAME-BASED TO LOVE-BASED

EMOTIONAL BALANCE

*"Everyone has his faults which he continually repeats:
neither fear nor shame can cure them."*
Jean de La Fontaine

Before I entered recovery, most of my decisions were based in shame. I felt shame for feeling my pain—something I could do absolutely nothing about. My decision to handle my pain through the use of opioids was based on this shame as well. Granted, my addiction may have started out with a legitimate need for pain relief, but it eventually evolved into something destructive. It was easier to face the day with the medication rather than facing my feelings without it. More drug use led to more shame, which led to more pain, which led to more drug use; the spiral went only one way—down.

I looked at my addiction to pain medication as a moral failing, my pain as a physical failing, my inability to communicate with others as a spiritual failing, and my feelings about the whole situation as an emotional failing. I felt tremendous shame and fear—neither of which was of any help in "curing" my faults. For that I needed love.

In pain recovery I restore the balance of this so-called failure. I work on these four areas individually, but collectively they support me in living a life based on love rather than a life based on shame.

*I choose to live a love-based life rather than a shame-based life,
because I know that in so doing I'm not only maintaining balance,
I'm having a life worth living.*

ADDRESSING THE WHOLE PERSON

SPIRITUAL BALANCE

....

"Chronic pain is a manifestation of imbalance, typically
physical, but also mental, emotional, and spiritual."
Adapted from Pain Recovery: How to Find Balance
and Reduce Suffering from Chronic Pain

In the book *Pain Recovery*, I learned that pain isn't the whole problem
and the absence of pain isn't the whole solution. I know that even if a
miracle occurred and suddenly my pain was gone, everything would
not be fine. There is more to the picture. I would still need to deal
with the damage caused to myself and others because of my chronic
pain. Even though I would no longer feel physical pain, I'd still need
to get into and stay in physical shape by exercising and eating well.
My thought process would still need to change and my emotional and
spiritual condition would still need to be tended to as a result of my
experiences with chronic pain. I would still need to be careful of my
dependence on medication, because it developed into more than a
physical dependence for pain relief, and became an emotional,
mental, and spiritual dependence as well.

If that miracle occurred, and I were suddenly rendered pain-free, unless
I continued to address my thoughts, feelings, spirituality, relationships,
and behaviors, the *only* thing that would have changed would be the
cessation of the physical pain. And today that is not enough. Today I
address the whole person. Today I address "all of me."

*Physical pain is only a small part of the big picture. Today
I understand that addressing the issues beyond just the physical pain
is what makes the difference between abstinence from medication
or absence of pain and pain recovery.*

LETTING GO

RELATIONSHIPS

....

"They simply embrace a gentle and benevolent manner of living in a world rife with hatred, bigotry, and man's inhumanity to man."
A Day without Pain

I'm changing the world around me. I'm doing this by changing myself. I do this every day that I stay clean. I do this with every step I work. I do this with every meeting I attend. I am learning to live in a world that doesn't always operate from spiritual principles by practicing spiritual principles. I don't expect others to practice these same principles; I am only concerned with my own recovery. So when I practice acceptance, forgiveness, or tolerance, I do so without expecting that others will understand or behave the same way in return. I let go of trying to control other people—I let go of even having expectations of other people. I release the need to change the way others interact with me or with each other. I embrace recovery. I embrace a way of life that is all about practicing principles.

I've found a way to be in the world that accepts others the way they are. I embrace the principles of recovery and allow others to live out their own lives. I'm not working a pain recovery program to change others, but to change the way I relate to others. I find freedom and the ability to love others when I let go of my expectations of others and leave what I cannot control to my higher power. I am only responsible for my actions today.

BABY STEPS

SPIRITUAL BALANCE

"Little by little, one walks far."
Peruvian proverb

While it is vitally important to begin and continue the work of recovery, and to do so diligently and consistently, it is also important to remember that when I was a baby, I crawled before I could walk, and I walked before I could run. There is a progression to all accomplishment, and I will approach my recovery with greater confidence and ease if I remember to take baby steps. I don't bite off more than I can chew today, or set unrealistic goals in my recovery. I do it little by little—but I do it!

I make progress toward balance, doing a little for each of the four points every day in order to change my experience with chronic pain. I make progress by remembering all the different things I can do today to help maintain my balance. I don't become impatient; I do what I can today, and I do a little bit more tomorrow.

ADVERSITY

MENTAL BALANCE

·····

"Adversity has ever been considered the state in which
a man most easily becomes acquainted with himself."
Samuel Johnson

When I'm faced with adversity, my natural response is to avoid it
at first, then to think about it until I simply cannot think about it
anymore. The downward spiral of thinking about problems usually
only makes the problems worse. I start creating problems that didn't
exist before I was faced with the initial adversity of getting through
a day or performing a particular task while in pain.

The downward spiral that I face in my mind when I am dealing
with adversity can be offset using the principles of recovery.
I make myself move, exercise, perform my routines, breathe,
pray, meditate, and reach out to others in my support group.

*When I face adversity I allow my mind to focus on the solution. I focus
on what I need to get done for my pain recovery and allow the other
"problems" I am facing to be worked out later. If problems remain after
I have done what I needed to do for my recovery, then at least I
can look at them with a clear head.*

SHAME AND GUILT

EMOTIONAL BALANCE

"Shame is pride's cloak."
William Blake

Shame says I'm no good; guilt says I've done bad things. Society would be a chaotic place if neither shame nor guilt existed; both are necessary human feelings that help us curb our more selfish behaviors. But sometimes shame and guilt can grow within us to the point that they cripple us and prevent us from living joyful lives in recovery. To feel either of these emotions to an extreme is, by definition, to be out of emotional balance.

Like everyone else with or without chronic pain, like everyone else in or out of recovery, I have done things I feel ashamed of; I know I am guilty of behaviors that have hurt others. Sometimes the shame and guilt I feel create so much pain that they threaten my recovery. I am grateful today that I have a solution in the Twelve Steps that allows me to address and make amends for the shame and guilt I feel over my past. Working with a sponsor, I can rid myself of toxic shame and guilt by working the steps and living a life in recovery today.

I can accept that I feel shame inside for who I am; I can accept that I may feel guilty for what I do, but I do not need to live in these feelings anymore. I work the steps and attend to my pain recovery program because I know there is something better than living a shame-based life.

STAYING IN THE MOMENT

SPIRITUAL BALANCE

"A number of approaches to spirituality emphasize the
value of staying in the moment, that is, being present-
centered in this moment, right here and right now, as
opposed to focusing on what has already happened in
the past or could potentially happen in the future....
I can neither change the past nor predict or control the
future. The only aspect of time and experience that
I have influence over is this moment, today."

Adapted from Pain Recovery: How to Find Balance
and Reduce Suffering from Chronic Pain

There are many ways in which staying in the moment promotes
health, healing, and pain recovery. In being present-centered and
living just for today, I make myself genuinely physically, mentally,
emotionally, and spiritually available. Helpful techniques to stay
in the moment and live just for today include concentrating on
and deepening my breathing by paying attention to inhaling
and exhaling; focusing on five to ten things in the immediate
environment, i.e., the room around me—walls, furniture,
ceiling, etc.; and meditation and prayer.

*I stay in the moment and practice getting into the moment by focusing
on some things around me throughout the day, noticing things I may
not usually notice—plants or flowers outside, equipment in an office,
traffic around me when driving in a car. Centering myself by taking
note of my immediate surroundings in the present moment helps me
ease into prayer and meditation, which promote spiritual balance.*

DILIGENT PRACTICE

RELATIONSHIPS

"Anyone with chronic pain can live more fully
as he or she learns to cultivate mindfulness, stress
reduction, acceptance, and positive regard. These
skills are developed like muscles and will eventually
replace the old, worn-out beliefs of 'poor me,' 'it's
never going to get better,' and 'I can't do it' that
many with chronic pain live with. Practice these
diligently and your life will change."
Adapted from Pain Recovery: How to Find Balance
and Reduce Suffering from Chronic Pain

Seeing others recover gives me hope. But hope without action is
just daydreaming and wishful thinking. As the old folk saying goes,
"If wishes were horses, beggars would ride." I don't need to beg for
recovery. It doesn't come to those who need it or wish for it;
it comes to those who work for it. It is good to get hope from
seeing people who have recovery, but only because I see what
they are doing and practice that as well.

Getting hope from others gives me motivation to do the things I
need to do for my recovery. I summon hope to break through the
resistance of laziness, procrastination, and distraction. I draw hope
from others to help during the dark and painful times. When in the
grip of loneliness, pain, fear, shame, guilt, and anger, I get hope from
others in my support group that there is light at the end of the tunnel.

*I put one foot in front of the other to get out of the tunnel I'm in. Those
in my support group offer me hope: the light to help me find my way.*

STRENGTH

PHYSICAL BALANCE

"Spirit has fifty times the strength and staying power of brawn and muscle."
Mark Twain

The human mind is capable of great things, but it's hard for it to focus on two completely contradictory states at the same time, for example, pain and joy. When I focus on my pain, then my awareness of it heightens. I feel the pain more intensely. Focusing on my pain gives it strength. But if I focus on the parts of my body that are not in pain, I make them stronger, and deprive my pain of the focus it needs to grow.

Focusing my physical actions on things that make me happy actually trains my mind to direct me to activities that will help my physical pain. Every time my pain starts creeping into my thought process, I make a conscious effort to take a physical, positive action. When my thinking is wrong, I focus on physical balance as a source of strength.

When my body is causing me physical problems, I focus on mental balance, because I know my thinking affects my physical pain. It might be as simple as remembering to focus on what I can do rather than what I cannot do. If my pain is in my back, I think about the strength I have in my arms and legs, for example. This is accentuating the positive, and strengthening my body through positive reinforcement.

I increase my strength by focusing my thoughts on my physical strengths. When my mind, body, and spirit are in pain and feeling weakened, I focus on the parts of my mind, body, and spirit that are strong.

AMENDS

MENTAL BALANCE

"The first step toward amendment is
the recognition of error."

Lucius Annaeus Seneca

I have learned that making amends is more than saying "I'm sorry."
Every day that I live a life without the use of medications to handle
my pain I'm making amends to myself and others for the damage
I caused as a result of my pain. I think about the life and recovery
that I have and remember that each day is a living amend.

When I forget about living my amends to myself and others, I open
myself up to the possibility of a relapse or regression. I give pain
the opportunity to take control of my life. I open myself up to the
option of considering the use of medication to manage my pain.
Instead, I look at the daily routine I have established as an amend to
everyone in my life and to me. I make it part of my practice to call
to mind the healing that is happening with more than just my body,
within all the relationships in my life, as a result of the healthy
choices I am making for myself and others.

I remember and call to mind that everything I am doing in my
recovery is a form of amends to myself and others. I honor the work
I do throughout the day and remember what others have done to
help me get to where I am and the price I have had to pay,
making sure it is not in vain.

MOVING ON FROM MISTAKES
EMOTIONAL BALANCE

....

"When you make a mistake, don't look back at it long.
Take the reason of the thing in your mind and then
look forward. Mistakes are lessons of wisdom. The past
cannot be changed. The future is yet in your power."
Hugh White

I may feel guilty because I didn't exercise or meditate or go to
a meeting, when instead I just sat around or let my day get so out
of whack that I ran out of time. I feel guilty later at night because
I could have, should have, would have, if only. When I find myself
in those "could, should, would, or if" conversations with myself,
then the odds are that I'm feeling guilty.

I may be feeling guilty because I had the choice to do something
positive and chose another path. Today I have several ways of
dealing with this guilt, but it starts with acceptance. I accept that
I made a choice I now regret, and move on from there. In the
future, I may do something different, something better, something
that demonstrates I have grown.

The awareness of my motivations and behaviors, which I have today as
a result of pain recovery, helps me avoid guilt and shame in the future.

*As long as I don't choose to use instead of dealing with and feeling my
feelings, every day is a successful day. Rather than feel guilty about
what I do or not do, I look at what makes me feel good and what
doesn't. I choose to move toward things that make me feel good and
loving rather than things that feed on my internal shame.*

TRUST
SPIRITUAL BALANCE

....

"Fear secretes acids;
but love and trust are sweet juices."
Henry Ward Beecher

Many people in chronic pain feel betrayed by the one thing they thought they could always trust: their own bodies.

Like many in chronic pain who have become addicted to pain medications, I sometimes feel betrayed by the medical profession; after all, the drugs that were prescribed to help ended up causing terrible problems. So how can health care professionals be trusted?

The list of culprits who eroded my trust can be extended *ad infinitum.* But all the finger-pointing in the world won't change the fact that in order to recover, I must practice trust. I can start by trusting myself—trusting that I have the inner resources to undertake this task. I can trust my higher power. I can trust the members of my twelve-step fellowships, who stand ready to help with their experience, strength, and hope. I can trust that if I follow the program of recovery laid out in my fellowship, I can recover, just as others have before me.

I can learn how and when to trust others. By continuously working a pain recovery program I not only learn to trust others, but I gain the trust of others as I become trustworthy myself.

LOVE

RELATIONSHIPS

"Love is about seeing people or ideals for what they actually are and embracing and supporting that reality. Love is expressed differently, but is the same across different relationships."
Of Character: Building Assets in Recovery

I can't be in spiritual balance without love, and love can't go forth from me unless I'm working toward balance. The extension of myself for the betterment of another, and accepting that others also want my betterment; my caring and nurturing of another spirit and accepting care and nurturance in return—these are all expressions of love. The extension of love may come in the form of listening, talking, a warm embrace, or a hand raised saying *no* or *stop*, setting a boundary. Love is not euphoric; love is what follows euphoria. Spiritual balance is not ecstasy; it is the calm *after* the storm.

Love is what I feel and practice toward myself and others after *the ecstasy and euphoria. My dedication to spiritual balance is love, a love that radiates from my dedication to achieving balance of spirit with myself and another.*

ADVERSITY
PHYSICAL BALANCE

....

"Smooth seas do not make skillful sailors."
Unknown

If life itself were always smooth and easy, we would never need
to develop the attitudes, abilities, and habits that serve us in times
of trouble. When these times of adversity arise, as they do in the
course of every life, not just in the lives of those in recovery, I can
use them as opportunities to build my character, and to strengthen
my program of recovery.

My higher power's will for me is not always easy to discern,
especially in times of adversity. Sometimes I become discouraged
and frightened, and I think about giving up. But if I have faith in
the tools of my program — prayer, meditation, service, connection
to my sponsor and others — then no matter how long it takes, I can
come through adversity with my recovery and my sanity intact.
Even better, I'll have experience under my belt that I can use
to help another in recovery when they feel discouraged by
adversity in their own lives.

*Every life contains adversity. I may not be the creator of the adversity
in my life, but I can choose to make it better or worse. Continuing
to work my program of recovery through adversity makes it better;
neglecting my recovery makes everything much worse. No matter what
life throws at me, I choose to pay attention to my recovery.*

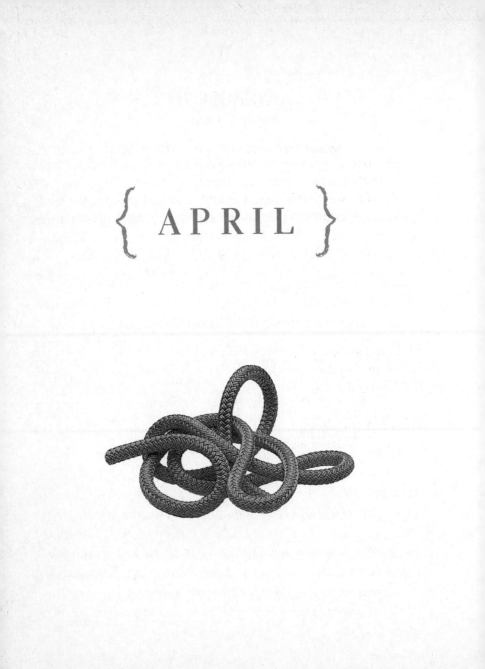

{ APRIL }

APPRECIATION

MENTAL BALANCE

....

"Good men and bad men differ radically.
Bad men never appreciate kindness shown them,
but wise men appreciate and are grateful. Wise men
try to express their appreciation and gratitude by some
return of kindness, not only to their benefactor,
but to everyone else."

Siddhartha Gautama, the Buddha

When I feel gratitude, I express appreciation. The mental process of expressing appreciation uses my thoughts and actions to show others that I feel grateful.

Making a gratitude list every evening helps me realize that even in the worst of times, I do have things to be grateful for. Perhaps it's just having the strength to hold a pen, or light by which to write, or the fact that I am literate enough to write and read. If I make the effort to think about it, and I am honest with myself, I will see that there is always something to be grateful for.

Of course, I thank my higher power every day for the gift of recovery. That is the thing I appreciate the most in my life today; from it flows all the other things I am grateful for.

I make the effort to show my higher power and others in my life that I appreciate all they do for me; I make words like "thank you" part of my daily vocabulary, and I think of what I have to be grateful for every day. Doing so takes my mind off my pain and puts it on my recovery.

LONELINESS AND ISOLATION
EMOTIONAL BALANCE

"Loneliness breaks the spirit."
Jewish proverb

As I read in *Pain Recovery*, loneliness is often a problem for those
with chronic pain because the onset of acute pain triggers an
automatic response that pushes a person in pain to withdraw from
society and "lick his or her wounds." Perhaps during mankind's
earliest days, it was adaptive to isolate and rest when sick or in
acute pain. Problems arise today because chronic pain appears
to stimulate this same desire to isolate, and ongoing long-term
isolation ceases being adaptive and becomes a source of imbalance.
It's too easy to fall back into old behaviors when I'm alone. I need to
make an effort to connect with others if I am to remain in recovery.

*Today, I have numerous ways of adapting to any pain or illness other
than by withdrawing from the human race. I don't need to become
cranky and rude, or push people away and so create my own loneliness
and isolation. I can let others know how I'm feeling, and I can be alone
without feeling lonely—I can choose to spend time by myself today,
and I can also choose to rejoin others and make a positive
contribution to their lives, as well.*

MEANING IN LIFE

SPIRITUAL BALANCE

*"The great art of life is sensation,
to feel that we exist, even in pain."*
Lord Byron

Like most people, I have a tendency to ascribe the meaning in my life to material things—the right job, the right car, the right house in the right neighborhood. Material things can make life more comfortable and pleasant, but they can never fill the void inside me. They may distract attention from internal emptiness or fill some of it temporarily, but such holes can only truly be filled from the inside.

Since chronic pain caused so many changes to my material life, it's been difficult at times to remember that the inner me hasn't changed. When I neglect who I am in favor of attending to what I do or what I have, my focus is outside of myself. I miss the meaning of life because that meaning and purpose come from within.

I begin to see that the true meaning in my life comes from spiritual balance; it does not and cannot ever come from material objects, no matter how beautiful or expensive.

I review the meaning of life for me—who I am rather than what I do and have. I take these thoughts through my day and focus on things in terms of the value they bring to my life. The most valuable things, I usually find, are those that are not material; they are spiritual: life, love, friendship, family. These are the true things of value in my life.

FAITH

RELATIONSHIPS

....

"Faith without works is dead."
James 2:14–18

My relationship with my higher power is based on the faith
I discovered in Step Two. That faith gave me comfort at a time
I needed it very badly; I would almost say it saved my life. But
faith alone will not keep on saving me in recovery—no—what
I need are work and service, because the old proverb is true:
"Faith without works is dead."

When my pain becomes great, or when my disease of addiction
starts eating at me, and when I think I don't have the ability to cope
with it without using or acting out, I call on the support system that
exists outside of me. I express my pain, my fears, insecurities, anger,
frustration, and so forth, in positive ways by talking or journaling
them out, not by acting them out. And I'm usually reminded that
the internal relationship with my higher power, my spiritual life, is
strengthened like a muscle when I get through another day of pain
by helping another person. It's amazing how this simple activity not
only gets my mind off my own problems, but also strengthens my
faith in my higher power, keeping me safe in recovery.

*The more I work the steps of pain recovery, and the more I get out of
myself and help others, the stronger my belief becomes in my inner
spiritual connectedness to my source of power—my higher power.*

RECOVERY

PHYSICAL BALANCE

"In recovery, we learn...about being responsible by listening with an open mind to our sponsors, other recovering friends, and family. We do our best to seek and consider their experience, strength, and hope."

Of Character: Building Assets in Recovery

Medications did not work for me anymore. I increased my dosages of medications to the point where they weren't effective. Doing that actually made my pain worse. The only thing that has worked successfully for me thus far has been my pain recovery program. Recovery doesn't mean the pain is gone; it means I'm living with the pain, managing the pain the way the doctors tried to do with medication. So when my pain increases, it's more important than at other times to listen to others in my program, to follow directions, and to remain disciplined in my program of pain recovery.

During times of pain, I do a little extra for my recovery, not a little less. I listen to those who have gone before me, benefiting from their experience, strength, and hope, and know that the program that worked for one person will work for another, if I work it.

ATTITUDE
MENTAL BALANCE

....

"The strongest principle of growth lies in human choice."
George Eliot

Attitude is a state of mind. I am free from addiction to
medication, and my mind is not clouded the way it was before.
With that clarity of mind I have the ability to choose how I
am going to express myself today, how I will act and what kind
of attitude I will have. Of course my life will always have its
challenges, but I do not need to add to the problem by having a
negative attitude. I always have my chronic pain to deal with, but
the way I choose to look at it on any given day is up to me. That
is the power and freedom I have in pain recovery.

I have the ability to decide how I'm going to respond. I have the
ability and tools to deal with what happens. Even in difficult and
challenging times, my pain—whether physical, emotional, mental,
or spiritual—can be lessened when I have a better attitude.

This takes time and practice. I will not always live up to my
own expectations for my attitude in recovery, but I have the ability
to think clearly enough to change the way I act with others.
This attitude is reflected with my friends and family, my
employment, my recovery, my life.

*I am conscious of my attitude and remember that I have the
choice and the freedom to think the way I want about the things
that are going on in my life.*

ACCEPTANCE OF LOSS

EMOTIONAL BALANCE

....

"Serenity comes when you trade
expectations for acceptance."
Unknown

Acceptance does not mean approval. Acceptance of significant
loss does not mean that there is no longer any distress related to
it. Losses that are fully accepted can still be painful, but they no
longer create serious emotional imbalances that hinder health and
healing. This is discussed in the book *Pain Recovery*.

Mourning for my lost health or physical ability and then healing
from that grief is a process of regaining balance, which takes
time and is different for each individual. This healing process
requires allowing myself to fully feel all the uncomfortable, painful
emotions that are part of saying good-bye to, and letting go of,
people and things that were important in my life. I accept my
losses with grace and dignity, and remember I still have
much to be grateful for.

*I remember that my pain is in inverse proportion to my acceptance.
I do the next right thing today, and let my higher power handle the
results. That is the way to serenity for me today.*

SELF-CONNECTION/CONNECTED TO SELF

SPIRITUAL BALANCE

"With spiritual balance I'm connected to the way I think and feel, and how I take care of my body. When balanced, my spirituality enhances my life. I do positive things that make me feel good, and I help others. I'm in harmony with the world and those in it. Whatever life brings, I'm able to deal with it and know that I'm okay. I'm able to find meaning and purpose even in situations that are painful and not to my liking. I live in and accept each day as it comes, changing myself instead of trying to change others."

Adapted from Pain Recovery: How to Find Balance
and Reduce Suffering from Chronic Pain

For me, a balanced spiritual experience includes certain characteristics. These include accepting myself and my place in the world, having a sense of purpose in life, being open to being challenged and even changing my beliefs, having a sense of inner strength on which I can draw, and having the following: values, beliefs, standards, and ethics that are mine and that I embrace. Perhaps most important, I have an awareness and an appreciation of a transcendent dimension to life beyond self, and a connection with that dimension, with what some may call God/Spirit/the Divine. I have a connection with nature, too, and I access this transcendent connection through regular spiritual practice.

I notice the things I'm doing in my life to maintain spiritual balance. Where I'm not doing these things I make an effort to do them, and where I am working on things to maintain balance I am grateful for those actions.

AMENDS

RELATIONSHIPS

"The real fault is to have faults and not amend them."
Confucius

In my active disease, I took and did what I wanted when I wanted, no matter whom it hurt. I was frequently dishonest and resentful, treating others as "less than," or as objects to be used to further my own ends. After all, I was in pain! I justified my actions to all who would listen. Today I see that in my disease I often acted out of my character defects, or what might be called my faults.

Today I have a program and a process for treating my defects of character, and it is in the Twelve Steps. I work on making amends to those I harmed in my addiction, and in so doing I amend my spirit. There is no shame in having character defects; they make me human. The shame would be in not amending them.

I make amends with the guidance of a sponsor, and know that there is no shame in doing so. What would be a shame would be to continue to live and act in my defects of character, hurting others along the way. I am vigilant today about my actions, and when I am wrong, I freely admit it. I make amends.

RESPONSIBILITY

PHYSICAL BALANCE

....

"At times it may be difficult to recognize we are
making a choice. We may try to avoid responsibility
by delaying a decision until we have fewer and fewer
options then tell ourselves, 'If only I'd known then
what I know now, I could have….'"
Of Character: Building Assets in Recovery

Should I take this class or that class? I don't know what teachers I'll have or what the course load will be like, so I do nothing. The devil is indecision. But I have to remember I can always change my mind. Recovery gives me that ability.

I find it's easier for my recovery and makes things go much smoother if I just make a choice and accept responsibility for that choice. If I don't like it, then I can change my mind later. But sitting and waiting until I make the perfect choice or feel absolutely right about doing something is a choice in itself. It's a choice to do nothing. The devil also finds work for idle hands.

I make a choice and have the freedom to change my mind. I take responsibility for my health by moving forward.

CATASTROPHIZING

MENTAL BALANCE

"The secret of health for both mind and body is not to mourn for the past, nor to worry about the future, but to live the present moment wisely and earnestly."
Siddhartha Gautama, the Buddha

I focus on the here and now instead of worrying about future calamities. I strive to avoid thinking about what has not yet occurred and to live in the moment. By remaining present-centered, I discover that nothing is as bad as I think it is. I do not allow my emotional catastrophes to affect my physical challenges. Through identification and awareness of my emotions, I do not allow potential catastrophes to run my life. I come to accept that my higher power and I can handle whatever is going to happen to me today.

Everything that might, could, would, or should happen is fantasy and imagination. If a catastrophe does happen, I accept that I can't actually change the catastrophe, but I can work on my reaction to it. I accept feelings about it and replace the thoughts of fear, such as worry, anxiety, or concern, and focus on recovery.

I strive to live a life free of needless worry and to reduce my stress level by not catastrophizing. I owe myself the opportunity to recover and to live a happy and healthy life.

DEPRESSION, SADNESS, GRIEF AND LOSS

EMOTIONAL BALANCE

"Going through multiple medical procedures or
treatments without noticeable benefits can add to
feelings of depression. These losses characteristically lead
to feelings of hopelessness, helplessness, and worthlessness.
Depression is sometimes described as anger turned inward
against oneself. If drug dependence or addiction to
pain medication is added to the picture, the severity of
these losses and the feelings that go with them typically
increase, creating further imbalances."

Adapted from Pain Recovery: How to Find Balance
and Reduce Suffering from Chronic Pain

Unresolved grief can contribute to both increased pain and drug
use. Although grief is a completely natural reaction to loss, the
more emotionally important the loss, the greater the grief associated
with it, and the more threatening it may feel to one's recovery.
Healing from grief involves the principle of acceptance. Mourning
or grieving refers to the process of saying goodbye to, and letting
go of, what I have lost. What am I grieving today? Is it the loss of
mobility or functioning caused by my pain? I may even grieve the
loss of pain medications, which may have come to seem like my
best friend, lover, and reliable confidant. I must remember that no
pain lasts forever, not even the pain of loss.

*I take a look at my unresolved grief and loss, knowing that no matter
how long I'm in recovery, I am always facing it in one way or another.
As I stay in recovery I feel things on a deeper level, and this requires a
heightened commitment to my program of recovery.*

UNTROUBLED
AND TRANQUIL

SPIRITUAL BALANCE

"A happy life consists in tranquillity of mind."
Cicero

Serenity is one of the first things I heard about in recovery, but it felt like the last thing I experienced. I actually started to feel it long before I could identify what it was. Many recovery fellowships read some form of the Serenity Prayer at meetings, and many members use this prayer throughout their days.

Serenity generally means a state of being *untroubled* or *tranquil*. Before pain recovery, I was not serene. I was troubled by my pain, troubled by those who did not understand, and troubled by medication that seemed to make my pain worse. In pain recovery, I found others who understood my pain and who did not judge me harshly. They accept me for who I am and have taught me that I deserve a calm and untroubled life. I know with the help of the fellowship, my sponsor, and my higher power, all things are possible.

I take the steps necessary to accept the things I cannot change, just as it says in the Serenity Prayer. Practicing acceptance and working on balance, I feel untroubled and tranquil, and can know peace. I strive to gain a greater understanding of serenity and to make it a part of my life.

ACTIONS

RELATIONSHIPS

....

"Well done is better than well said."
Benjamin Franklin

I used to talk, talk, talk, if only to myself, about my "problems."
Rarely did anything get done. If I had a difficulty in a relationship,
my first thought would be "I'd better spend some time alone,
analyzing this problem. That's how I'll get to the bottom of it."
Today I know better than to try to solve a problem with the same
thinking that created the problem. Today I know that the
antidote to my disease is action.

Action may consist of prayer and meditation, reading recovery
literature, attending a meeting, working with a sponsor or a
newcomer, or being of service to someone else, whether they are
inside or outside of my recovery fellowship. Getting out of myself
and into service to another is the best way for me to "work on"
my relationships today.

*Today I know that the solution to my difficulties is in action. Any
problems with my relationships with others can be helped, not by
morbidly dwelling on problems, but by taking action to get out of
myself and into service to others. When I forget this, I'm grateful that
I have a fellowship that reminds me of what I need.*

WILLINGNESS

PHYSICAL BALANCE

....

"It appears that some part of the feeling or motivation
of willingness is a gift and outside our control."
Of Character: Building Assets in Recovery

It's nice when I get out of bed in the morning refreshed,
rejuvenated, invigorated, and motivated to face the day.
And that's the way it really is, some days.

On other days, recovery can be exhausting; there is so much to do.
I must remember to pray and meditate, attend meetings, exercise,
think of others, work with a sponsor—it takes energy I
sometimes don't think I have.

I rejoice in the days when I do feel motivated, excited, and
energetically charged to do the tasks that lie ahead. I consider these
days a blessing of courage and strength from a higher power. On
every other day I ask for *willingness*. And usually, it comes.

*It's easy to be an angel when no one is ruffling my feathers. I practice
willingness to improve my physical balance and well-being by doing
those things for my recovery that I may not want to do. I embrace them
with the same enthusiasm I have for things I do want to do.*

ACCEPTANCE

MENTAL BALANCE

....

"Nothing is a greater impediment to being on good
terms with others than being ill at ease with yourself."
Honoré de Balzac

Acceptance of physical pain is the beginning of pain recovery.
To resist pain is to give it strength and continue to let it have power
over my life. In pain recovery I accept my chronic pain. In essence,
I'm making friends with my pain because it is a part of me. As I
progress through my recovery, I build a stronger relationship with
all the various parts of me. I become more at ease with myself.

Acceptance, a key principle of recovery, does not come
immediately, but over a period of time. It requires a renewed
commitment on a regular basis. It is normal to think, "I don't want
to be in pain." It's normal to want to avoid pain, whether physical
or emotional, or to fantasize about a life without pain. In recovery,
however, I can't afford the luxury of such fantasies. I continue
to become aware of these thoughts and desires through prayer,
meditation, writing, and attending meetings. I accept that I have
them and then replace negative thoughts with thoughts
of recovery—which is the solution.

*Pain doesn't keep me down or prevent me from being whole. I may not
be able to do everything I once did, but I am complete, a beautiful part
of my higher power. I accept that some pain is inevitable, a necessary
part of life, and an opportunity to grow.*

DEALING WITH LOSSES

EMOTIONAL BALANCE

"The feelings of sadness, grief, and loss are closely related to one another and often fall underneath the umbrella of depression.... Sadness, grief, and even symptoms of depression seem at times to accompany my chronic pain. When my pain became a constant companion, I began to suffer significant losses, including my ability to work and physically function as before, the ability to participate in previously enjoyed recreational and family activities, financial losses, and hopes and dreams for the future."

Adapted from Pain Recovery: How to Find Balance and Reduce Suffering from Chronic Pain

Coping with these varied emotional states is easier when I remember to use the tools of my program: prayer, meditation, journaling, exercising, and sharing with others.

When the feelings of grief, loss, sadness, and depression hit—and they do, at times—I do not wallow in them. Instead I think about how far I've come in my life in recovery, and realize I have much to be grateful for. The more I focus on what I can do and the actions I can take for my pain recovery, the more emotionally balanced I become.

MANY PATHS OF SPIRITUALITY

SPIRITUAL BALANCE

"Feeling confused or ambivalent about spirituality is understandable.... My challenge here is to be open to the possibility that growing a relationship with a power greater than myself is a dynamic key to learning to cope with life in ways that are balanced, healthy, and helpful.

There is no single path on a spiritual journey. In order to find the path that is right for me, I may travel many roads to get to where I need to go. On those roads are many guides that help me along the way. Spirituality is not so much about answers as it is about learning how to appreciate the journey itself. The essence of spirituality is that it's an ongoing quest for learning and fulfillment."

Adapted from Pain Recovery: How to Find Balance and Reduce Suffering from Chronic Pain

Spirituality is what I make of it today. I seek connectedness with my higher power, as I see others in my fellowship doing. I believe that what works for them will work for me, too. I may feel unsure or even a little foolish at first, but with practice, the answers come.

I am open to the many paths of spirituality, knowing that if what I'm doing is not working for me, I have the freedom to explore other avenues. I also know that I get to take what works for me from all sorts of different paths—recovery is a personal process.

FORGIVENESS

RELATIONSHIPS

"Pray you, now, forget and forgive."
William Shakespeare

In recovery I learn to accept that the people in my life have done the best they could do, and I forgive them for the times they have disappointed me, remembering that, at times, I have disappointed others and need forgiveness, too. Some people in my life have disappointed me by not being more understanding of my pain, others by just not being there for me enough.

When I practice acceptance of the shortcomings of others, I realize that maybe the things I classify as shortcomings are not that at all; maybe I have had unrealistic expectations of others—maybe the other people in my life really have tried to do their best in relation to me. Maybe that's what I need to accept, and forgive. And maybe in the future I need to practice living without expectations, which seem only to arouse resentment in me when they are not met.

I forgive everyone in my life, I pray for them if they are not present and in my life currently, and I hope for the best for them. I seek to have empathy and understanding. I do all of this because it actually helps me in my own recovery and in my ability to handle my chronic pain.

I ask my body to do the best it can to carry me through this day, and help me be of service to others. The same forgiveness I give my own body I give to others today as well, knowing that just as I have limitations, so do they.

TIME TAKES TIME

PHYSICAL BALANCE

....

*"Time means different things to different
people at different moments. For shuttle astronauts,
the ten seconds before blastoff are awe-inspiring.
During a heart attack, milliseconds equal a lifetime.
For some kids, the last hour of the school year
seems to go on for weeks."*
A Day without Pain

Some days are just easier to get through than others. The first hours of not abusing medication felt like an eternity. Today, it feels like an eternity since I last used medication abusively.

I do not participate in the downward spiral of addictive thinking by placing value on the time it has been since the last time I thought about using, or the last time I actually used. What matters is that I do not use medication abusively, no matter what— the amount of time since my last use is less important than the quality of my recovery.

The only relevance time has to my recovery is the strength that I build and the foundation I stand on with each day I put together without abusing medication. But time does not mean that the thoughts and obsessions will go away. During the times when seconds seem like a lifetime, I pray. And when time flies by and my recovery feels strong, I pray.

SUMMONING THOUGHTS
OF KINDNESS

MENTAL BALANCE

"Our lives are full of opportunities to be kind. How
often and how well we respond to these opportunities
will influence the quality of our own lives and the
lives of those around us."
Of Character: Building Assets in Recovery

When I'm in enough physical pain I may believe it's too much to
ask of me to actually extend kindness to others. Even a smile for
another is too much to muster sometimes. My friends, family, and
support group can understand when I'm in this level of pain, and
they take comfort in knowing that I'm in the pain recovery solution.
They do not fear that I'll revert to active addiction because they
get to watch me cycle through pain in a way I never could when I
was abusing medication. However, even during times of extreme
distress, I do have the power over my thoughts. Kindness starts with
my state of mind, and extends itself into action toward others.

*I think kindly of myself and others, summoning the strength from my
higher power to have kind and loving thoughts for others. I intervene
on negative, hateful, hurtful thoughts and replace them with thoughts
of kindness. Then I follow those thoughts through with action.*

RESENTMENT

EMOTIONAL BALANCE

....

"Resentment reinforces feelings of being victimized.
Feeling like a victim makes pain recovery more difficult
because victims don't take responsibility for their own
choices and actions. And today, in order to progress
in my recovery, I know I must take responsibility for my
choices and actions. I can't afford to wallow
in resentments. Fortunately, my recovery program
gives me tools and steps to take in order to keep
resentments from festering."

Adapted from Pain Recovery: How to Find Balance
and Reduce Suffering from Chronic Pain

Twelve-step programs have a marvelous mechanism for handling
and discharging resentments—the inventory process. The Fourth
and Tenth Steps suggest that when resentful, I pause and take an
honest look at my own part in things. When I am wrong, I admit it,
and stop finding fault with the person or persons I resent. Although
they may have wronged me, too, I don't focus on them. I keep the
focus on me—because I am the only one I can change.

*I talk about my resentments in an appropriate manner, as described
in the steps. I talk about them without yelling, screaming, threatening,
or acting out. I apologize when I am wrong, and most importantly,
I don't repeat my part in the behavior.*

SERENITY

SPIRITUAL BALANCE

"Descend still deeper into yourself, until you
hear nothing but a clear, undivided voice, a voice
which does away with doubt and brings with it
persuasion, light, and serenity."

Henri Frédéric Amiel

I had become so identified with my chronic pain that it
had become part of my core identity. This being so, I could
rarely experience serenity.

When I'm thinking of myself as a chronic pain "victim," it interferes
with my ability to maintain serenity. However, if I'm calm and
focused on my serenity, I'm less likely to have thoughts of being a
victim. This paradox—what comes first, the proverbial chicken or
the egg?—becomes less paradoxical over time.

Over time, I come to identify myself as more than just
my chronic pain, impaired functioning, or manifestation of
addiction. I identify myself with my level of serenity in spite of how
I'm feeling physically. I am strong. I am valuable to my loved ones
and to myself. I maintain a balanced sense of self that is essential
to my serenity.

*The most important thing in my life is my recovery, which is dependent
upon my level of serenity. When I'm focused on my serenity and
maintaining the four points of balance to support that serenity, then
all other areas of my life, including my chronic pain, are tolerable.*

SHARING FEAR

RELATIONSHIPS

....

"It requires strength and courage to do anything
that is uncomfortable or to do things differently from
the way you've done them in the past. Therefore,
rather than reflecting weakness, admitting to and
talking about your fears reflects strength."

Pain Recovery: How to Find Balance and
Reduce Suffering from Chronic Pain

I was once ruled by fear—fear of things that were likely to happen,
and fear of things that had almost no chance of ever happening. I
had no way to distinguish between healthy and unhealthy fears, or
between useful and destructive fears.

I know the difference today; there are, indeed, healthy fears. Fear
of crashing my car makes me drive with care; that's healthy. Fear
of catching flu during an epidemic makes me take precautions like
getting a flu shot and washing my hands frequently. Healthy fear
leads me to make healthy decisions.

Another example of healthy fear is my fear of relapsing—of my
returning to abusing medications to manage my pain. It's easy to
become paralyzed by this unhealthy fear—paralyzed into inactivity.
I can become so fearful of losing my recovery that I stop doing the
things I need to do to preserve it. But there is a solution: I can share
these fears with others in my support system, and then work through
them. I can participate in my recovery and lessen my fears.

*Fear shared is fear lessened. I take an honest look at what I'm afraid
of and share that with another person.*

FLEXIBILITY AND STRETCHING

PHYSICAL BALANCE

"Stretching exercises are used to help keep muscles and ligaments limber and flexible. Stretching can ease stiffness, increase your range of movement, reduce stress on joints, and increase the flow of blood and nutrients throughout the body, all of which can help you fight pain."

A Day without Pain

I continue to work on increasing my flexibility. It's easy to become complacent in recovery once I start to feel better. I must continue to work on my physical abilities or my body is susceptible to additional injury, just as my spiritual self will be susceptible to relapse if I stop working my recovery program.

Just as I continue to work the steps every day in order to keep my recovery strong, in pain recovery I take it a step further. I focus on my body as well.

Stretching and exercising on a regular basis keeps me physically prepared to handle what comes my way. It makes it possible for me to stay in recovery. If I don't stretch, keeping my body in shape to the best of my ability, I'm setting myself up to get injured and perhaps need medication. I'm setting myself up for a relapse.

Part of my ongoing recovery process is monitoring my physical flexibility. I make sure that I'm making progress in this area, checking in with my level of flexibility in a given area on a regular basis and being accountable to a physical therapist or someone in my support group with whom I work/exercise.

NONJUDGMENTAL

MENTAL BALANCE

···

"Acceptance, in regard to character,
is actively reaching out for an understanding
that suspends judgment in favor of better
knowing another person or ourselves."
Of Character: Building Assets in Recovery

Suspending judgment doesn't mean refusing to judge. It means
withholding judgment until all the facts of a case or situation can
be considered. Many in our society have come to consider all forms
of judgment bad, wrong, or even cruel. "You're being judgmental"
is spoken as if it's an insult. But how are we to discern the right
course of behavior for ourselves if we don't use judgment?

Good judgment is necessary for us to make informed decisions.
However, in order to make intelligent decisions, judgment must
be based on a full examination of issues. Withholding judgment
until all sides have had a chance to present their points of view is
simply the intelligent way to make decisions, especially in matters
as important as my recovery.

Others may come to different decisions for themselves; only after
hearing them out and evaluating their decisions in light of my own
recovery can I make an intelligent judgment.

*I accept the way others think today, focusing more on the destination
than the roads on which we traveled.*

A P R I L

27

ANGER

EMOTIONAL BALANCE

....

"What can I do about anger? First and foremost, awareness that I'm angry is necessary in order to make a conscious decision as to what to do about it. It is helpful to ascertain what I'm really angry about—the true reason that I'm angry. Knowing the source of my anger and looking beneath the apparent reason to a deeper level is valuable in examining my emotional reaction.

The next steps in dealing with anger are identifying my wants and needs related to what's happening; selecting the solutions that are the best fit from the available options and then taking actions to implement those solutions. This solution-oriented process provides a direct route to finding balance and consequently turning down the volume of my pain. I can look at the most recent instances when I was angry. I look at what happened to my pain level when these situations occurred. By looking at the underlying emotions in these situations, I can discover different ways of getting my wants and my needs met."

Adapted from Pain Recovery: How to Find Balance
and Reduce Suffering from Chronic Pain

Anger is neither good nor bad; it is an emotion that has its uses, but more often than not represents wasted energy. I cannot afford to waste my precious energy today.

I am aware of anger as a reaction to not getting my perceived needs met. However, today I realize that in recovery, my needs are always met; it's just my wants that sometimes go unmet.

MEDITATIONS FOR PAIN RECOVERY | 129

SELF-IMAGE, SELF-ESTEEM, SELF-CARE

SPIRITUAL BALANCE

"You may have become so identified with your
chronic pain that it becomes part of your core identity;
you may begin to think of yourself as a 'victim,'
and pain becomes who you are rather than an
experience that you sometimes have."

Pain Recovery: How to Find Balance and
Reduce Suffering from Chronic Pain

The progressive nature of my chronic pain and addiction led
me to be less able to do the things that I once did with ease.
Ongoing use of opioids and other medications led to impaired
thought processes. As this took place, over time, my self-image
and self-talk became increasingly negative and focused nearly
exclusively on my losses and deficits. This happened gradually
enough that I was unaware of the changes in my thinking and
consequently in the way I felt about myself.

I am not defensive about this today. Instead, I am willing and able to
admit to myself and others how badly I may be feeling about myself.
I do not overcompensate or try to be perfect at the things I can do.
I do not withdraw or stop trying. I continue to take care of myself—
which is an ongoing process. It is possible for me to have a "normal"
life today, even though there are times when I may not feel like I can.

*I look at my abilities, my limits, and what matters to me. This is part of the
process of change and leads me back to balance when I'm out of it, keeps
me in balance when I'm in it, and helps me live the life I want to live.*

HONESTY

RELATIONSHIPS

....

"That my heart has once again opened is the gift of
recovery. In my active addiction, I lived in so much pain.
I was always afraid of being hurt and feeling the kind of
pain I recently experienced."

Tails of Recovery: Addicts and the Pets That Love Them

The healing power of honesty never ceases to amaze me.
When I am brave enough to be honest, opening my heart to
another and letting him or her see me as I am in all my frailty,
I am putting my faith not in that person or his or her reaction,
but in my higher power, and in the knowledge that my higher
power will always provide the love and security I need, even
if the people around me cannot.

If my honest feelings are angry, I do not lash out and justify it by
calling it "getting honest." I have healthy ways to get honest that
don't hurt myself or others today.

*I take an honest look at the things that make me angry and resentful
and share those in a constructive way with my sponsor or support
group so that I can find a solution.*

EXERCISE

PHYSICAL BALANCE

"One of the primary problems with
chronic pain is the lack of movement to protect
or 'splint' the places that hurt."

Pain Recovery: How to Find Balance and
Reduce Suffering from Chronic Pain

Through exercise I can maintain a healthy weight, increase my flexibility, build strength, increase my serotonin level, and protect and strengthen my heart and circulatory system, as well as increase dopamine levels that improve my mood and energy.

The more I exercise, the greater my tolerance level becomes to the exercise itself and to my pain. Where once I could only move a little, I now find that I can tolerate much more. As a result, even when I'm not exercising, I find that my tolerance level for pain has increased greatly and I don't need to use drugs to increase it.

I continue moving, stretching myself just past the edge of my comfort zone, knowing that in doing so I'm increasing my tolerance for pain and my capacity for healing.

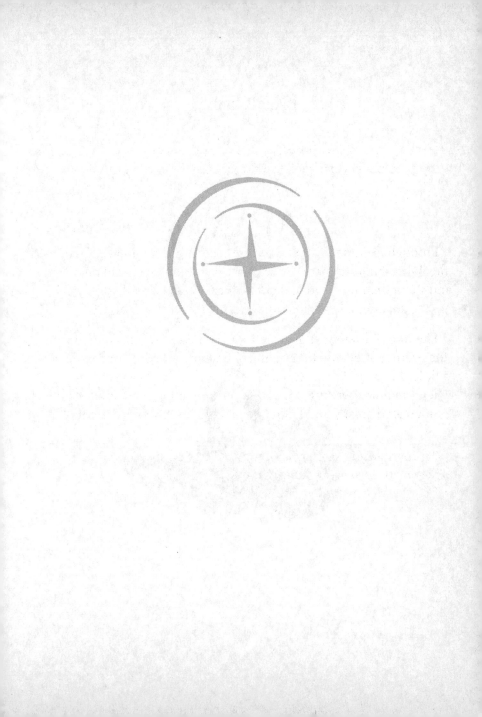

{ MAY }

RESPONSIBILITY

MENTAL BALANCE

"Being responsible is a very demanding character asset. It requires that we know ourselves and own our choices and the consequences of those choices. Being responsible means knowing what things in life are in our control and focusing our attention on those things."

Of Character: Building Assets in Recovery

I take responsibility for my pain recovery by focusing my thoughts on those things over which I have control, like the number of meetings I go to or the doctor appointments I make. I have control over exercise, eating well, and also how I behave and act toward my friends and family when I'm in pain. I have control over how often I pray and meditate. I have control over the writing and reading I do.

I do not have control over other people or over my chronic pain, only my relationship to them. I monitor my thought processes regarding the things I have control over. When I catch myself thinking too much about things over which I have no control, I redirect my thoughts to thinking about my pain recovery program, to thinking about a higher power, to constant prayer if that's what is needed.

I take responsibility for my recovery by accepting that there are things over which I have control. I focus my mental energy there and leave the rest to a loving higher power and the world to figure out. I'm only responsible for my relation to that world, not for what is in it.

SECONDARY EMOTIONS

EMOTIONAL BALANCE

"In most circumstances, anger is really a secondary emotion. It often forms immediately and automatically (this happens unconsciously, so there may be no awareness of it) in response to a situation that brings up feelings of hurt, fear, and/or inadequacy. Hurt and fear are the primary emotions that anger covers up.

Anger serves several defensive purposes. It works as a shield that deflects uncomfortable primary emotions so they can be avoided or kept at a distance. Anger provides a sense of power and control, and directs focus outward to identifiable, external scapegoats. It is almost always easier and more comfortable to focus on the actions of others than it is to focus on myself."

Adapted from Pain Recovery: How to Find Balance and Reduce Suffering from Chronic Pain

As I drove along one day, a car zoomed up and passed me, almost clipping my fender. I became enraged, and began to chase after it, when I realized that for a split-second before I became angry, I had become afraid. That helped me see the relationship between fear and anger. I realize that anger is often just a secondary emotion, and I can feel and then set aside my fear instead of lashing out in anger.

I allow myself to experience the vulnerability of revealing the underlying, core feelings I'm experiencing and don't mask those feelings with anger. I'm aware I almost always play a part in the problems I experience.

PEACE

SPIRITUAL BALANCE

"Peace comes from within. Do not seek it without."
Siddhartha Gautama, the Buddha

When I think of peace, I think of a declaration between two warring parties that hostilities are over and issues are finally settled. But even with peace, often there is tension remaining, and confusion about how those two sides will interact with one another in the future. There is still an uncertainty about the future, rebuilding to be done, and some unsettling quality to those coming back from war and returning to what was a normal life before that war. Peace does not mean the work has ended. In many ways, peace means the fighting has ceased and the real work is only just beginning.

My chronic pain and my desire to fight it were at war. My desire to fight it needed to win at any cost, to be rid of the enemy (pain) and wipe it from the face of the planet.

The treaty that has been signed is my commitment to recover. But just because the war is over does not mean the work has ended; in fact, the peace between these warring sides of my body and being is just beginning. My spirituality, my quality of life, hangs in the balance. The ongoing building of my spiritual fitness is like the negotiations of the terms of peace.

I acknowledge that peace is not a state of being, but a process, and requires work. I put work into the "peace process" that is my recovery, my acceptance of my chronic pain, and returning back to a life that is forever changed, a landscape forever altered by the war that has been waged against myself.

CONTROL
MENTAL BALANCE

....

*"Fear less, hope more; Eat less, chew more;
Whine less, breathe more; Talk less, say more;
Love more, and all good things will be yours."*
Swedish proverb

In recovery I actually have some control over life. The part I control is my relationship to life, the thoughts I have about life, the actions and feelings that follow, and in the end, my spiritual condition, which improves as a result of my thoughts and actions. Good thoughts and good actions lead to good results.

I used to believe that what I *thought* was who I was. However, the more I live life without medicating my feelings, the more I realize that nothing is further from the truth.

While my thoughts are part of me, they are only a part of a much bigger picture. There is a separation between my self and my thoughts. I became so identified with my thoughts that I believed there was no separation—until I started working a First Step. Then I learned that I might not have control over the first thought, but I had control over the action that followed. I began to discover that action then talked back to the thought, thereby changing the thought.

When I think and act out of love, my life is truly filled with more of the good things that I need for my recovery. I have no control over my life's events—the only thing I control is my reaction to them. When that reaction is positive, then so is my life.

EMPATHY AND FAMILY

RELATIONSHIPS

"Empathy for a loved family member in chronic
pain is not something we can turn on or off. When we
love the person in pain, we want to do whatever we
can to help stop the pain, or at least make
it as bearable as possible."

A Day without Pain

It's hard for me to really understand what my family goes
through when I am in pain. But the longer I stay clean and in
recovery, the more I appreciate the pain my friends and family
experienced (and still do) when I'm suffering from chronic pain.
Today I realize that just as they empathize with those feelings,
they also feel the benefits and joy of recovery.

The more I recover, the more my loved ones get to feel that joy as
well. The longer I stay clean, the more motivated I am to handle
my own feelings so they don't have to. I use the steps, meetings,
therapy, a sponsor, prayer, meditation, reading, and writing as just
some of the ways to process my feelings so that I don't carry them
home to make my family handle them.

*My family and friends can feel my rage, shame, fear, guilt, anger,
and loneliness when I'm not processing those feelings in a healthy way.
When I am in recovery and working through my feelings, they can
feel my joy. I give my friends and family the joy I deprived them
of in my active addiction.*

STRENGTH

PHYSICAL BALANCE

....

"Dwell not upon thy weariness; thy strength shall
be according to the measure of thy desire."
Arab proverb

There are many kinds of strength. Physical strength is my ability
to endure and cope with my pain. Mental strength is my ability
to accept pain as a necessary part of everyone's life, including
mine. Emotional strength is my ability to handle my emotions in a
healthy way that hurts neither myself nor others. Spiritual strength
is my ability to find a power greater than myself, a transcendent
dimension to life that gives me the capacity to continue my
recovery in the face of my physical pain.

All these areas of strength are important, and interdependent.
I do what I need to do today to maintain my physical strength,
including eating right, exercising as my condition permits, and
getting adequate rest and hydration.

I pay attention to the areas of my life that are important to me,
and today, my physical strength is important. I may not be as
strong or as flexible, or have as much endurance as I once did,
but I cherish what strength I have today, and do what I need
to do to preserve and protect it.

*Without physical balance, I may become unbalanced in the other
important areas of my life, with a resulting diminishment of my
recovery. That is not the outcome I want today. Today I seek balance
and serenity in all areas of my life, including the physical.*

DIRECTING ANGER

EMOTIONAL BALANCE

"Anger is the emotional response to things that don't go the way I want them to. Anger results when I feel I've been wronged in some way. Depending on the situation, anger is a healthy and appropriate reaction. Problems with anger usually occur in how this powerful feeling is expressed.

Anger can be expressed along a broad continuum— from suppression, which can raise my blood pressure and create emotional and physical discomfort in my own self, to explosive expression, which can lead me to hurt or abuse others. Anger...can cause significant stress and...increased muscle tension and increased pain."

Adapted from Pain Recovery: How to Find Balance
and Reduce Suffering from Chronic Pain

When I'm in pain I may feel anger at people close to me whom I perceive as not understanding or being supportive enough, or at the doctors I blame for being unable to help or for prescribing the medications that I became addicted to. The list of targets for my anger is long, unless I begin to practice acceptance and realize that other people are not here to meet my needs. My higher power is intimately involved in every area of my life, and my job today is to accept the will of that power and to tap into its strength when I'm in pain or in anger.

I accept that anger is a natural response to frustration and pain. I ask my higher power to help me accept situations I cannot change, and focus on serenity rather than catastrophe.

IMPATIENCE

SPIRITUAL BALANCE

"Time is not a cure for chronic pain, but it can be crucial for improvement. It takes time to change, to recover, and to make progress."

A Day without Pain

As a person in recovery, I know only too well what it feels like to be so impatient that I think I can't stand waiting one more minute. Impatience is one of my character defects—I want what I want when I want it, which is usually a few minutes ago! How can I be expected to take the time necessary to practice the principles and steps of recovery? I'm willing to try, but it takes so long... I know that a pill or a shot is not the answer for me today, but boy, either one would sure work fast, and bring me the kind of relief I *think* I need.

When I'm impatient and my recovery process seems too slow, I ask my higher power for patience, willingness, and courage to do what I know is healthy for me, even when I'm so impatient that I don't think I can stand waiting any longer. My higher power has never let me down.

It takes time for the pain to pass. Anything real takes time. Recovery is a lifelong journey, not a pit stop. I can be patient, knowing that time will pass, and so will my pain, as long as I practice my program of recovery.

ALIENATION FROM GOD/ SPIRIT/HIGHER POWER

RELATIONSHIPS

"Twelve-step fellowships have demonstrated, over many decades with millions of people, that the concept of coming to believe in a power greater than oneself is an essential part of the process of recovery. The same principle applies to pain recovery."

Pain Recovery: How to Find Balance and Reduce Suffering from Chronic Pain

All those who seek conscious contact with a higher power, whatever that power is called, experience periods when they feel that contact intensely. This contrasts with periods when people may feel absolute alienation from that power. Spiritual writers have referred to the two differing feelings as consolation (heightened contact) and desolation (lack of conscious contact).

Early in my pain recovery, I imagined my higher power as a sort of spiritual Santa Claus, responsible for making me happy or sad by giving or withholding his favors. Thinking this way, it was easy to feel, when in adversity, a sense of alienation from my higher power—the state of desolation. It took time for me to realize that even when I am not getting my own way, my higher power is taking care of me, and always has been. At times like these, when I realize that even in adversity my higher power cares and provides for me, I feel consolation. I feel secure in my personal relationship with God/Spirit/higher power today.

I have a relationship with my higher power that is personal and my own; however, like every relationship in my life, it requires time and attention. If I'm feeling alienated from my higher power, I have the ability and freedom to be closer.

LOSS

PHYSICAL BALANCE

....

"Suffering is the individual's response to a
painful stimulus. It is unique and it involves emotions.
We all suffer sometimes in our lives, whether it is physical
or mental or emotional or spiritual or a combination
of all of these. Aristotle and Plato insisted that suffering
(pathos) is a necessary part of the human condition.
More than 2,500 years ago, the Buddha taught in
his 'Four Noble Truths': 1. Suffering exists. 2. Suffering
arises from attachment to desires. 3. Suffering
ceases when attachment to desire ceases.
4. Freedom from suffering is possible."

A Day without Pain

Chronic pain was a deeper level of suffering than I'd ever
experienced. Now that I'm free of pain medication, even with
chronic pain under some control, I get to deal with the human
condition—which, as the word "human" implies, affects everyone.
This is not a new concept, but the idea of my using the Twelve
Steps as a way to heal the suffering I've always experienced in one
way or another is a revelation. I participate in recovery, not only
so I can be free from abusing pain medication, but also to
heal the relationships in my life.

*Life is full of suffering, and chronic pain can be salt
on an already-existing wound from simply living in the human
experience. But freedom and diminished pain are possible
through working the Twelve Steps.*

SERVICE

MENTAL BALANCE

....

"How can I be useful, of what service can I be?
There is something inside me, what can it be?"
Vincent van Gogh

I admit it—the last thing I want to do when I'm feeling bad is to be of service to anyone or anything. I don't see how the solutions to any of my problems are going to come from helping another person, getting to a meeting early or staying late to help clean up, or doing a little something extra to help around the house. I often think, "I'll do that later or when I'm feeling better." However, the truth about chronic pain is that I'm never going to feel completely better—sitting around and waiting to feel better only got me addicted to pain medication and destroyed most of my relationships.

I've learned in pain recovery that first, I stop using the medication and take positive action—and *then* I feel better. Being of service is a necessary part of any recovery program, and in pain recovery it is especially important. Service not only gets me out of myself, it helps others and it also gets me out of my head, even if just for a moment. Every moment that I'm of service, thinking of someone or something other than myself, I'm not thinking about my chronic pain. When I'm not thinking about my pain, then I'm not making it worse than it already is.

Today I act and serve in a way I would "if only" I were feeling better. I take action today and leave the "if only" in the hands of a loving higher power.

ANXIETY

EMOTIONAL BALANCE

....

*"Fear not, but trust in Providence,
wherever thou may'st be."*
Thomas Haynes Bayly

Anxiety is a major cause of increased pain. Anxiety can be thought of as low-level fear. It can be defined as distressing uneasiness, nervousness, or worry felt in response to any situation I anticipate to be threatening. It is usually accompanied by doubt about my capacity to cope with it. Some of the physical symptoms of anxiety are sweaty palms, increased heart rate, muscle tension, breaking out in cold sweats, inability to sit still, and/or a feeling of being uncomfortable in my own skin.

A large percentage of people who have chronic pain report experiencing elevated levels of anxiety. An effective way to decrease my anxiety is by learning and practicing relaxation and self-calming skills such as meditation, deep breathing, progressive muscle relaxation, guided imagery, self-hypnosis, and even quiet downtime. Balanced individuals experience manageable levels of appropriate anxiety. A holistic approach is most effective in helping me develop healthy habits to continue practicing in order to establish the emotional balance that enhances my pain recovery.

I practice effective, healthy habits to decrease anxiety, such as reducing caffeine intake, paying attention to nutrition, staying in the moment, meditating, reading recovery-related material, exercising, paying attention to spirituality, practicing yoga or Chi Kung, or exploring Reiki.

DOING THE FOOTWORK

SPIRITUAL BALANCE

....

"Consider the lilies of the field, how they grow; they
neither toil nor spin, yet I tell you, even Solomon in all his
glory was not arrayed like one of these."
Matthew 6:28–29

My program of recovery teaches me that my higher power does
for me what I cannot do for myself—this means that there are
certain things I can and should do for myself as a responsible, self-
supporting person in recovery. I do "the footwork"; God handles the
results. This philosophy helps me accept that although I must take
right action, the results are not up to me—and isn't that a relief?

When I take an honest look at my life, I begin to see that just as
God created the beautiful lilies of the field, He also created me.
He created me, and He provides for my needs, provided I do the
footwork. After all, I'm no lily—I am a human being in recovery.
I can and do take responsibility for my life today, and rely on my
higher power to do for me those things I cannot do for myself.

*I take responsibility for my spirituality today. My understanding of
it is constantly evolving in pain recovery. Like any of the four points
of balance, with spiritual balance I may swing from one extreme to
another. In pain recovery I examine, remember, and cultivate my
relationship with my higher power.*

EXPECTATIONS

RELATIONSHIPS

"Have faith that no matter what happens, you will be okay. You may not get exactly what you want, but perhaps, to your surprise, you may get what you need."
The Soul Workout: Getting and Staying Spiritually Fit

When I least expect to feel an inner connectedness to a higher power is usually when I "get" it. As in so many other external areas of my life, my internal, private relationship with my higher power surprises me. My expectations are not always met in the ways that I anticipate.

My higher power works in ways I don't always expect; and although my prayers are always answered, often the answers come in forms and ways I could never have predicted. (And that's okay, because what I expect often falls far short of what my higher power has planned for me.)

When anyone, from my higher power to my next-door neighbor, behaves or reacts to me in a way I didn't expect, I can easily become resentful. And resentment is harmful to my recovery. Instead, I accept that my higher power has a plan for me, and that no matter what happens, it will be better than anything I could have expected.

These days, I try to live in acceptance rather than anticipation.
I accept; I try not to expect.

DISEASE OF ADDICTION

PHYSICAL BALANCE

"Becoming addicted to painkillers is the manifestation of a disease. It is a disease of denial, and for some people who have a prescription problem, they just don't realize it or want to admit it."
A Day without Pain

Addiction manifests in many ways: drugs, alcohol, gambling, sex, shopping, work, love—even codependency, or addiction to another person.

Addiction is pervasive. It is not a moral question. It is not a choice. It has nothing to do with the substance, behavior, or thought process *per se*. It is a physical process that occurs in the addict's brain, which has spiritual, emotional, and physical implications.

Today I understand that addiction has little to do with a substance and more to do with a process. I see my addiction manifest in many different ways once I stop abusing medications. I must continue in recovery, or I see rather quickly and painfully how my disease will find other things to latch onto in order to take me out of myself and give me relief, albeit temporarily. Surrendering to the knowledge of my addiction is much deeper than just not abusing pain medication.

I have a disease. Abusing pain medication is only a symptom of the disease. I continue working steps on the disease because once the pain medication is gone, my disease will find other ways to manifest.

SERENITY
MENTAL BALANCE

....

"Worry gives small things a big shadow."
Swedish proverb

My thought process has a direct relationship to my serenity level. If I allow my thoughts to go unchecked, they create a negative spiral that leads to toxic shame, guilt, fear, anger, and pain. In pain recovery I have a choice: I can intervene on the toxic, negative thoughts as soon as I'm aware of them, as quickly as possible.

I tell myself to stop and make room for serenity. Today I know that thinking leads to behaving, and behaving leads to feelings, and feelings have a direct effect on my physical well-being, and my ability to live another day without abusing pain medication and acting out in a way that really only increases my pain.

When I'm not feeling serene, I can change that by correcting, interrupting, and stopping the thought process that leads me in that direction. When I find that I'm "powerless" and can't control my thinking, I call on my higher power, who helps me, sometimes through people in my life: my recovery fellowship, sponsor, therapist, or counselors.

I think of serenity, monitor my thoughts, and intervene on those thoughts that move me away from serenity.

ACKNOWLEDGING FEAR

EMOTIONAL BALANCE

"Fear not for the future, weep not for the past."
Percy Bysshe Shelley

Fear can be difficult to acknowledge to myself and others. Having lived with physical and emotional pain for a long period of time, I learned to suppress my fear. I don't like to admit to or talk about being fearful. In some circles, feeling scared and expressing fear may be viewed as weakness, making it even harder to discuss with others because of the desire to avoid negative perceptions and judgments. My family and friends may view my expression of fear as a sign that I'm relapsing in my pain recovery. They may get scared themselves and react negatively to my talking about fear, thinking that I'm not being positive.

Acknowledging fear requires strength and courage. It takes strength and courage to do things differently today from the way I've done them in the past, and acknowledging fear is different for me today. I do it not to gain pity or attention, as I may have done in the past, but to bring it out into the light of day where it often shrivels and loses its power over me. Rather than reflecting weakness, admitting to and talking about my fears reflects strength. I keep in mind that courage is not the absence of fear; courage is being aware of my fear and doing what I need to do in spite of my fear.

I acknowledge my fears and remember that courage is not the absence of fear, but being aware of my fear and taking the actions necessary for maintaining my emotional, mental, physical, and spiritual balance.

POWERLESSNESS

SPIRITUAL BALANCE

....

"Once members in the program admit their
powerlessness over drugs or alcohol or food or sex or
gambling or whatever obsession in which they are
engaged, they are free to begin the recovery process.
This type of admission opens the door for acceptance."
A Day without Pain

The process of admission of powerlessness over my disease and
my pain is not a one-time deal. I admit my powerlessness daily,
and use all the tools at my disposal—prayer, meditation, reading
recovery-related or inspirational literature, attendance at meetings,
working with a sponsor and others in recovery, and being
of service—to help me overcome both my pain and the disease
of addiction, which I know will always be with me even though
its manifestations may be kept at bay.

Admitting powerlessness keeps me in spiritual balance because it
helps me realize I am not in control; my higher power is. As long
as I keep myself spiritually fit and in balance, my higher power will
never give me more than I can handle. I admit my powerlessness
and ask for help, and it always comes.

*I accept my circumstances relating to pain. I turn negatives
into positives by admitting my powerlessness and remembering
that when I admit, accept, and stop resisting or trying to be in
control, I decrease my pain.*

SOLVING FAMILY PROBLEMS

RELATIONSHIPS

"Many family troubles linked to chronic pain can be solved by being open and honest. Problems generally develop over time and only escalate because members try to avoid acknowledging them. Communication is a two-way street and involves not only expressing what you are feeling and getting others in the family to see your point of view, but also listening to others and really trying to understand what they are experiencing."

A Day without Pain

Communication is important, especially between my higher power and me. In prayer I talk to my higher power, and in meditation I listen for my higher power. The answers always come, if I am open-minded and willing.

Lack of communication with my higher power leaves me with few resources to help in my recovery. I become snappish and cranky with those around me, especially my family, and communication between me and my loved ones becomes strained, if it occurs at all.

I remember that communication is a two-way street, and I share my thoughts and feelings with others, making sure I listen to them, because they have needs, too.

Before I communicate with others, I communicate with my higher power. I make sure my primary relationship is the one between my higher power and me. That relationship is the one that makes all others possible. Being right with my higher power helps me in my relationships with everyone else.

DEPRESSION

PHYSICAL BALANCE

"The likelihood of a person taking pain medication to relieve the depression associated with or caused by unremitting chronic pain is significant. Recent studies reveal that the rate of major depression is directly related to the amount of pain a person feels; the greater the pain, the more likely there also will be symptoms of depression."

A Day without Pain

At times I still wonder why I'm feeling depressed. I need to remember that pain recovery does not mean instant healing. I still need to live with the pain and the implications of that pain, which can include depression.

I remember today that I'm developing tools in my program of recovery that help me handle both my pain and any accompanying depression. Through following that program, I don't give the depression more power than my pain. I go about the routines of my life and accept that some days I feel depressed, but I don't necessarily need to dwell in it. I exercise, even lightly; meditate or even briefly share with another, even slightly; and recover, one more day.

Just like my chronic pain and addiction, I'm powerless over the symptoms, such as depression, on any given day. However, as for my chronic pain, I have a solution that includes actions, steps, and a program I can work so that I don't need to stay depressed for any longer.

PATIENCE
MENTAL BALANCE

"Experience has taught me this, that we undo ourselves
by impatience. Misfortunes have their life and their
limits, their sickness and their health."
Michel de Montaigne

"Slow is real." I heard a woman say that once in a recovery meeting,
and it stuck with me. As a person in recovery, I understand very well
what it means to want what I want when I want it (and then want
more of it); but today, with the tools of my recovery program, I'm
turning impatience to patience, one day at a time.

When I sit still and attentively through an entire meeting, I'm
practicing patience. When I wait my turn in the supermarket line,
I'm practicing patience. When I listen while someone else shares,
I'm practicing patience. All this mindful practice helps me become a
more patient person, which is so different from the way I used to be,
always impatient for the next thing that I thought would "fix" me.

Patience is an aspect of serenity and one of the gifts of recovery;
it comes slowly, but when it does it stays with me, and makes
it so much easier to get through my bad days, and it makes my
good days better, too.

*It takes mindfulness to train myself to be patient. It may not
be second nature yet—but that's something that will come, too,
in time; I can be patient while I wait for patience to become a
working part of my nature.*

FEAR

EMOTIONAL BALANCE

....

"Fear is the thought of admitted inferiority."
Elbert Hubbard

When I feel fear, often it's because I don't believe I am enough—
that I am not good, smart, or strong enough to handle whatever life
might throw at me. I need to realize that my higher power created
me the way I am, and that is enough. I'm no better and no worse
than anyone else. I am enough. And not all fear is bad.

Fear is a natural human emotion that can help me to respond
effectively to things that might harm me, like walking out into the
middle of a busy highway—that kind of fear is protective. Fear
becomes a problem when I allow it to debilitate me by keeping me
from doing the things I need to do in order to function in the world.
I can also allow myself to be troubled by fear about something that
might happen, but that probably never will—anticipating the worst.

Fear feeds on itself; the more fearful I am, the more fearful I
become, and the less able to function. The antidote to fear is faith—
faith that tomorrow can be better than today, faith that my program
of recovery, which has worked for so many others, will work for me,
faith in my higher power, faith that I can succeed in my recovery.

*I acknowledge that many if not all of my fears spring from the fear of
the unknown, or fear of change, or fear that I am not enough. Faith is
the antidote to my fear. When fear threatens to overwhelm me,
I remember: The more fear, the less faith. The more faith, the less fear.
I know which I prefer to live in today.*

INTUITION

SPIRITUAL BALANCE

"An under-recognized facet of spirituality is intuition.
Intuition is a conversation, hearing an inner voice that is
always there. Being intuitive is similar to common sense,
a subtle, underlying knowingness or understanding.
Intuition means actually hearing and listening to that
voice. It is not the voice in my head, but the voice deep
in my heart that tells me if I'm doing the right thing. It's
usually a quiet voice that requires practice to hear."
Adapted from Pain Recovery: How to Find Balance
and Reduce Suffering from Chronic Pain

In early recovery, I was unaccustomed to tapping into the source of
all my strength, my higher power, through prayer and meditation.
Now, however, I am used to seeking inner guidance, and my
thoughts and intuitions are frequently helpful to myself and others.

*I listen to that inner voice, trusting that it knows what is best for me. I
start with small things and know that the longer I stay in recovery, that
inner knowingness reveals itself in situations that are more and more
important in my life. I have the ability to trust myself—that's a big
difference from when I was addicted to pain medication.*

FAMILY "ORGANISM"

RELATIONSHIPS

"The family is a complex organism. And, like any
organism or system that has diverse parts that make
up the whole, it functions best when all the different
elements are in good working order."
Pain Recovery: How to Find Balance and
Reduce Suffering from Chronic Pain

Focusing on my own spiritual balance helps bring serenity to my
family. It might not fix everything, but at least by working on my
own spiritual balance I'm making a contribution to the family unit
and living in the solution, rather than contributing to chaos and
dysfunction, as I once did.

Addiction is a family disease. While it may be true that other
members of my family need to find their own recovery program,
I don't wait for them to find recovery before seeking recovery for
myself. My family is not responsible for my recovery, and I'm not
responsible for anyone's recovery but my own. But perhaps I can lead
by example if I keep my side of the street clean, take responsibility
for my own actions, contribute time and resources to the best of my
ability, and remain self-supporting. Today I make the principles of
recovery the guide by which I live with my family and friends.

*Addiction is a family disease. Recovery is a family healing process.
I bring recovery into my house today to banish and heal the damage
of the disease I brought in yesterday, for the hope of a joyful
and light tomorrow.*

UNDERSTANDING CHRONIC PAIN

EMOTIONAL BALANCE

....

*"Like feeling the burn from touching a hot stove
tells us to stop touching it, emotional pain is evidenced
so we will stop doing something, learn, grow,
and hopefully become smarter."*
A Day without Pain

Chronic pain is pain that has outlasted its original purpose of warning us of danger or telling us something is wrong for which we should seek treatment. Will I ever understand my chronic pain? I don't know. Is it important that I understand it? Maybe. Maybe not.

I do know that my program of recovery gives me tools to deal with both my chronic pain and the abuse of pain medication that it has caused. I don't need to understand either pain or addiction to benefit from working my recovery program.

Emotional pain has been present since my physical pain became chronic. Perhaps even before that. Today I know that my emotional pain is just as severe as the chronic pain that it is a reaction to. My recovery program gives me the tools to deal with both my physical pain and the emotional pain that accompanies it.

I have faith that I learn from my emotional pain because I'm in recovery today; I don't need to keep going through the same pain.

A PROCESS, NOT AN EVENT

MENTAL BALANCE

....

"It is not an easy reality to face, but just as your chronic
pain did not develop overnight, neither will the solution
to finding relief develop in a day or two."

*Pain Recovery: How to Find Balance and
Reduce Suffering from Chronic Pain*

My difficulties did not develop overnight, and neither will the
solution. This realization can be discouraging; I want relief and
I want it quickly. After all, I'm only human.

What is the solution, then? My mind clamors for relief, and my
thoughts can seem to work against me, until I remember to slow
down, to breathe, and to take the actions that my mind doesn't want
me to take when I am overwhelmed with my own pain. "Bring the
body, and the mind will follow," I remind myself.

I tell myself to move, to get out of bed; at first I resist, but I remember
the advice to "bring the body," and I take these actions. My mind
resists praying, or meditating, or reading recovery literature, but
I do it. I tell myself to attend a meeting or meet with a sponsor or
counselor in spite of how I feel, and I do so. I repeat this process every
day, for many days, and in time I am experiencing greater well-being
and more relief. Soon these actions become instinctive. I am working
toward my own recovery, slowly—but surely.

*I bring the body, and the mind follows. I have faith in the recovery
process, and faith itself is an action I take, training my mind to think
about such events or activities that will bring me relief and recovery.*

SENSITIVITY

EMOTIONAL BALANCE

"Emotional sensitivity can contribute to emotional imbalance. People who are emotionally sensitive feel things more rapidly and more deeply than others and tend to personalize them. Emotionally sensitive people may learn ways to numb themselves from their feelings because so many of their feelings are painful."

Adapted from Pain Recovery: How to Find Balance and Reduce Suffering from Chronic Pain

Am I any more or less emotionally sensitive than anyone else? That's hard to say—although chronic pain will give anyone a heightened awareness of his or her own pain. Whether or not I started out as an emotionally sensitive person, I accept that I have a heightened sensitivity today.

Being aware of this, and of my tendency to personalize painful events, I remember that painful things happen. They are not necessarily directed at me. "The rain falls on the just and the unjust," it is said, so when painful events rain down on me, I remember that "the rain" is falling on others, as well— it's not personal.

I realize today that it's okay to have feelings and to even be a little oversensitive sometimes, but now I don't have to let those overpowering feelings rule my life. I feel my feelings without labeling them or personalizing my pain.

AVOIDING FEELINGS

SPIRITUAL BALANCE

....

"Many with chronic pain have deliberately developed
a pattern of avoiding emotions. We do our best to
ignore and deny these feelings because they are so
unpleasant. They never go completely away, however.
In most of us, these feelings hover just out of sight,
casting a dark shadow of misery. They cause problems.
Often by ignoring them we are in reality allowing
these negative feelings free rein over our mood and
experience, and become a victim of the very thing
we are fighting not to have. We expend a lot of effort
attempting to avoid the things we label unpleasant,
undesirable, or unwanted. Again, the harder we
resist, the more we suffer."
A Day without Pain

I take responsibility for my feelings rather than avoiding them today.
I acknowledge them and honor them by turning them over to my
higher power, rather than running, avoiding, using, acting out, etc.
I pray and meditate, asking my higher power to take those feelings
from me and direct my attention to the next indicated action.
I ask for help and it comes.

*I take responsibility for my feelings today; in accepting rather than
avoiding feelings, I'm able to find spiritual balance.*

FLEXIBILITY

MENTAL BALANCE

....

"CBT (Cognitive Behavioral Therapy) encourages you
to realize that you must play an active role in your
therapy. You must be an active participant, and it is
imperative that you understand you can change the
pain. Once you stop believing you are a passive victim
in a situation over which you have no control, real
changes can and will begin to happen."

A Day without Pain

The belief that I must play an active role in my recovery is a change
in my thinking, and requires mental flexibility on my part. If I'm
flexible, or open-minded, it makes it possible for me to be more active
and frees me up to try different things: ideas, activities, friendships,
etc. Flexibility frees me in my relationships with others, too.

I'm flexible enough to give others' ideas a try. I'm flexible enough
to say, "You know, maybe I was wrong," or "I'm sorry." I go with
the flow or try something new. I listen to other people and become
flexible in my beliefs and ideas. I don't have to give up my
principles; I can just realize that other people have a right to their
opinions, and sometimes, those opinions are right.

I'm able to release my hold on my pain, freeing me to reach out to
a higher power, build a relationship with my higher self, and have
more freedom from pain in my recovery.

*I practice open-mindedness by being flexible, flexibility being the
action of open-mindedness.*

OPEN-MINDEDNESS

PHYSICAL BALANCE

*"Chronic pain is complex, with many different layers that
affect your mind, body, and spirit. It can be relentless and
poses a very real threat to living a full, vigorous life."*
A Day without Pain

There are many different aspects to chronic pain. Through pain
recovery I've discovered information about my brain, medications,
addiction, feelings and emotions, family, treatment, and spirituality.
I've explored the complicated nature of chronic pain and the
simplicity of recovery; I know now that recovery is an ongoing
journey, and I'm always looking forward to the next steps. I
continue to seek out holistic solutions and replace the thinking that
tells me I'm unable to do things without medication.

Through an ongoing commitment to recovery, my life becomes
one of wellness, balance, and restored function. Spirituality and
pain recovery require mindfulness and awareness, which means I'm
always in a state of exploration and discovery. What worked for me
yesterday may not work for me tomorrow, and likewise, what didn't
work yesterday may be tomorrow's solution. I'm always in a state of
open-mindedness, wonder, and exploration. I explore new, healthy
activities and therapies to deal with my chronic pain and physical
functioning in different ways.

*I am open to new solutions and, at the same time, I honor and
remember the power and complexity of chronic pain, knowing that
by definition it may always be a part of my life, and for that reason
recovery must always be a part of my life as well.*

POWERLESSNESS

MENTAL BALANCE

"There is potential for addiction in everyone
who uses narcotics, and just because you have
a prescription for opioids from a doctor doesn't
mean you are safe from addiction."

A Day without Pain

The hardest thing for me to do was surrender to the fact that I had become an addict and was using pain medication addictively. I knew people who were addicts from all walks of life and backgrounds. Some of them never used anything addictively before pain medication. Was I like all of them? Yes. I was an addict with chronic pain.

Once I admitted my physical addiction, I had to address the psychological, emotional, and spiritual implications of that addiction. I had to admit that the physical compulsion to use medication addictively was only one part of my problem; it had become an emotional, mental, and spiritual obsession and compulsion. Admission and acceptance have only made the process of recovery easier for me.

Admitting and accepting powerlessness is the first step toward accessing a higher power to help me live free of my addiction in recovery. Accepting my pain and addiction does not mean approving of either. I will continue to seek outside support from others in recovery.

I focus my mind on the concept of powerlessness, which means accepting and surrendering to my addiction, giving me the ability to act in humility about my disease and my recovery.

{ J U N E }

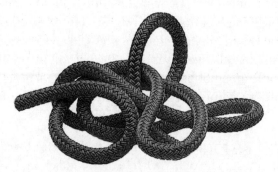

EXPRESSING FEELINGS

EMOTIONAL BALANCE

....

*"Most people struggling with chronic pain and
dependence on pain medication try to avoid
emotional as well as physical pain. Our common
thought process tells us that if we can just avoid the
pain, it won't affect us. However, in the same way
that lightning always finds a path to ground, feelings—
including painful and uncomfortable ones—always
find a path to expression."*
Adapted from Pain Recovery: How to Find Balance
and Reduce Suffering from Chronic Pain

Today I have a choice in the way I deal with my emotional and
physical pain. The choice is to address my feelings in the moment,
without further damaging myself or others, or to avoid my feelings
and overreact in uncontrolled, explosive ways. Allowing my painful
feelings to be expressed through my behavior only adds more
suffering to my life and the lives of others. Emotional balance gives
me the capacity to choose which path I take, instead of letting fear
and avoidance make the choice for me.

*Today I have the ability to choose the path my feelings will take,
instead of avoiding or ignoring them until they explode. I don't hurt
myself or others today by ignoring painful feelings; I look within myself
and use the tools of recovery to deal with them.*

POWER

SPIRITUAL BALANCE

··

"The power of our beliefs can transcend physical
conditions and often results in marked improvement in
our level of pain and certainly in the amount we suffer."
A Day without Pain

In active addiction I was completely powerless over my chronic
pain, and began abusing the medication I was given to "manage"
it; my resulting behavior reflected this powerlessness as well. The
irony is that since I've admitted powerlessness over addiction and
chronic pain, I've found some power just in knowing that I've
got a spiritual solution to my problems. The pain I feel is a little
more manageable, simply (or not so simply) as a result of having a
program and structure to follow and having other people in my life
who have been through the process, and who can serve as examples
to me that, in fact, the process does work.

*I've got the power to not be a victim, to live with my pain,
and to transcend my physical conditions; that power lies in the
process of recovery.*

WILLINGNESS

RELATIONSHIPS

....

*"Acting in willingness requires that we do what we know
to be right even when we don't feel like it."*
Of Character: Building Assets in Recovery

The more I do for myself, the more I build the relationship
between me and my higher power. It may not seem like a
traditional form of practice in spirituality, but I can dedicate
everything that I do throughout the day to that inner
connectedness needed to have a joyous life.

I show my willingness to be closer to my higher power by
showing up to my exercise class, by going to work and putting my
efforts into that task, by helping others, or even by doing the dishes
or my part of the chores around the house. I do these tasks willingly
and mindfully, and the relationship with my higher power
grows as a result.

This external practice of willingness can and does do more for my
internal peace and connection to my spirit at times than reading or
rituals. I work on my spiritual, inner life by practicing willingness
to do the things outside of myself that I may not *want* to do on any
given day, but I do them and dedicate myself to doing them well.

*I dedicate my external, more worldly tasks and activities to the inner
life, peace, serenity, and connection I long for.*

FEAR

PHYSICAL BALANCE

....

"He who fears being conquered is sure of defeat."
Napoleon Bonaparte

At times, my fear can overwhelm me. Perhaps it's the fear derived from the anticipation of pain. Perhaps it's fear derived from my insecurities in a given situation. Regardless of the fear's seeming origin, it creeps in insidiously, exacerbating my emotional and physical pain. Eventually, I become angry, defensive, or withdrawn because of this fear. Fear increases my pain and throws me into a state of physical imbalance. Fear, in effect, creates or worsens the very situation I fear.

However, when I'm centered and I take the time to contemplate my situation, I realize that through the guidance of my higher power, the fear begins to dissolve. I see through the illusions of physical and emotional pain brought on by fear. I set aside my fear of pain, and have faith that my higher power will carry me through my day.

The more I interact with my higher power, the more I come to rely on that power. The more I rely on my higher power, the less I fear.

CONCENTRATED EFFORT

MENTAL BALANCE

....

"It has been demonstrated by people at risk of
depression that by concentrated effort they can
change their brain chemistry, thereby reducing
their risk of depression."

A Day without Pain

In recovery, I do have the ability to change the way I feel. What I'm
powerless over is that first thought, the one that says that something
outside of myself—some chemical, behavior, or thing—is going
to change the way I feel. There was a time when I'd compulsively
pursue such a thought. But I'm in recovery now.

Recovery helps me gradually change the first thought that comes
to mind, until eventually, my first thought becomes something I
can trust in again. At first, I must really concentrate my efforts until
my thoughts have changed, but in time, my first thought will not
be of using or practicing any other unhealthy behavior in order to
change the way I feel. I may instead think first of practicing prayer
and meditation, of improving my conscious contact with my higher
power, or being of service to others. I rewire my brain, changing
it to something that produces healthy first thoughts, and I do this
through the process of recovery.

*I concentrate on recovery, steps, meetings, sponsorship, prayer,
and meditation. Through concentration it eventually becomes
second nature to do things for myself that are recovery-based and
will heal rather than harm.*

BODY-EMOTION CONNECTION

EMOTIONAL BALANCE

"Anger and resentment, fear and anxiety, grief and loss, depression and sadness, loneliness and isolation, guilt, shame, embarrassment, ambivalence and uncertainty, self-pity, serenity and peace, love, hope, gratitude and appreciation, compassion and empathy
...and others."

Adapted from Pain Recovery: How to Find Balance and Reduce Suffering from Chronic Pain

When I entered recovery, if you'd asked me to make a list of my emotions, it would have contained three items: happy, sad, and angry. That's a short list. But in recovery I've learned that I have many emotions, and many shades of each emotion. Sometimes I feel happiness tinged with sorrow or satisfaction colored by regret. What I know today is that I own my feelings; they do not own me. I need not be afraid to feel my emotions, unmitigated by the mask of addiction.

It is important for my pain recovery for me to remain in touch with all of my emotions and to know where they manifest in my body. I stay conscious and cognizant of my emotions and this awareness becomes a great tool for me, so that sometimes I can know how I'm feeling just based on what's going on in my body. Knowing what I'm feeling helps me stay on top of my recovery and provide myself with what I need.

I take the time to remember my emotions and where they manifest as feelings in my body. I make a list of my emotions, update my list, or reflect on the existing list as I pay attention to what I'm feeling physically and what that means for my recovery.

EXTREMES OF SPIRITUALITY

SPIRITUAL BALANCE

"If passion drives you, let reason hold the reins."
Benjamin Franklin

Extremes in any of the points of balance result in overall imbalance and interfere with the process of pain recovery. A spiritual extreme might consist of maintaining rigid, inflexible, set-in-stone beliefs that I have convinced myself represent the absolute and only truth. Most often, this attitude fuels a closed-mindedness that prohibits any actual examination of such beliefs and precludes openness to any other possibilities.

At this end of the spectrum, all other beliefs, forms of spirituality, or conceptions of God typically have to be rejected as false or inferior since my belief is the "one true way." Never mind that my best thinking brought me to the extreme worst state of my life, before I entered recovery—I must know best!

Actually, it's when I avoid extremes in all areas of my life, including spirituality, that my recovery flourishes. I don't need to become dogmatic, or a zealot, and I certainly don't need to set myself up as an authority or judge of other people and their spiritual growth. That is not the way of recovery.

I work on growing my spiritual life, and accept that I can find answers from others who may have different beliefs. That is how I learn and grow in recovery—there is no room to grow when I start out at an extreme. I want room to grow in my recovery, always.

MEDITATION AND PRAYER

RELATIONSHIPS

....

*"Blessed are the ears that hear the pulse
of the divine whisperer, and give no heed
to the many whisperings of the world."*
Thomas à Kempis

Meditation quiets the chatter in my head. I find that
practicing meditation eases my physical pain and helps me
in my recovery, which is what gives me the ability to engage
in healthy relationships as an equal partner, no matter what
my physical abilities or pain level.

The Eleventh Step describes the importance of using prayer
and meditation to build a relationship with a power of my own
understanding—a power that is greater than me. Practicing prayer
and meditation as a way to build a relationship with my higher
power teaches me the value of these practices in all areas of my
life, with everyone in my life. Listening is the key to healthy
relationships, with my higher power, and with others.

*I find a meditation technique that works for me and practice
it whenever possible. I can experiment with different meditation
practices I learn about from recovery program friends or from reading
books. Whatever works for me is the practice I use to build
a relationship with my higher power.*

ACTIONS

PHYSICAL BALANCE

"Let us rise up and be thankful, for if we didn't learn a
lot today, at least we learned a little, and if we didn't
learn a little, at least we didn't get sick, and if we got
sick, at least we didn't die; so, let us all be thankful."
Siddhartha Gautama, the Buddha

When I have a headache or a backache, or my chronic pain
feels intense, I feel like I can't possibly go to the gym, take a walk,
or even just move. After all, I'm not going to be able to perform
the way I used to, or the way I want to, anyway, so why bother?
However, when I follow the exercise regime I've established,
regardless of the way I'm feeling, I'm pleased to discover that
having motivated myself to exercise, even a little, I've experienced
a corresponding relief from pain. This lightens my mood
and my thinking, in an upward spiral of physical, emotional,
and mental balance.

Positive action is a powerful signal to the body. By taking positive
action I'm sending a message to my body that I'm in recovery today.
I don't push myself too hard, but I do push myself. I can't think my
way into a better way of living; I must live my way into a better way
of thinking. I do this by taking positive physical action in my life,
every day. I'm grateful for every small action I'm able to take today,
and that gratitude in itself makes my pain a little less.

*I take positive action. It can be something as simple as taking a
shower or bath, eating well, and making sure to exercise today within
the best of my ability.*

SANITY

MENTAL BALANCE

···

*"Our plastic brains change every time we learn a new
word, try a new activity, experience a new pain,
and every time we forget a name."*
A Day without Pain

Every new thought I think has the potential to change the actual
structure of my brain—that's a serious thought! In the past, of
course, I thought nothing of changing the structure of my brain
with substances or unhealthy behaviors; today, in recovery, I do my
best to introduce only healthy, uplifting, or supportive thoughts and
ideas into my brain. I want to alter my brain for the better now
that I am in recovery.

Everything—from the books I read to the prayers I say, the
meditation I practice, the meetings I attend, the movies I view, and
the people with whom I surround myself—is positive today, and
supports my recovery. I maintain my mental balance by introducing
only thoughts and ideas that will enhance my recovery.

*I take care of my brain with the things I offer to stimulate it, making
sure I'm seeing, hearing, and speaking recovery. I imagine that each
thing I touch, taste, smell, hear, or say is forever imprinted on my brain
and has the potential to either impart recovery or perpetuate pain.
Today I choose to live in recovery.*

DEVELOPING AWARENESS
EMOTIONAL BALANCE

....

"The capacity to identify, feel, and express my
emotions is essential to a balanced state. I may have
great difficulty, especially in the beginning, identifying
feelings and expressing them in ways that support
emotional balance. This difficulty is only magnified
by my chronic pain."
Adapted from Pain Recovery: How to Find Balance
and Reduce Suffering from Chronic Pain

There are several levels of awareness involved in cultivating
emotional balance. The first level requires me to become
consciously aware that I'm experiencing a feeling, an emotion.
Although I may not know specifically what the feeling is, it is
important to simply notice and acknowledge that I have some
feeling; I have been numbing myself for so long.

The next step is for me to identify what the particular feeling
is. An important part of identifying my emotions is to put them
into words. As an alternative to not knowing what I'm feeling or
feeling confused, it is helpful to label the feeling: *I feel anxious,*
or *I feel angry,* or *I feel depressed.* The more specific I can be in
identifying my feelings, the more likely it is that I will understand
the emotional experience.

*I'm pleased to be developing continued awareness of my
emotions. Recovery, and the awareness it brings, allows me to
notice and identify my feelings today, instead of blindly acting out
on feelings I don't understand.*

TRUST

MENTAL BALANCE

....

*"I know the plans I have for you, declares the Lord,
plans to prosper you and not to harm you,
plans to give you hope and a future."*
Jeremiah 29:11

I like to think of myself as an intelligent person who thinks clearly, yet it's true that my trusty thinking once told me it would be a good idea to abuse my pain medications. Now I know that trying to control my pain by abusing medication was a result of my thinking that I could control or manage my life, my way. When I stopped trying to manage my pain in this way, and instead entered recovery, learning to rely on a higher power, somehow things got better for me. My life was restored to sanity, and I learned new ways to manage my pain.

At times I still wanted to rely on my own thinking to help me in recovery; I thought I could judge which of the tools of recovery — meeting attendance, helping others, journaling, step work, etc. — I needed and which I could do without. Needless to say, until I started trusting in my higher power and the experiences of those in my recovery fellowship, I struggled. Today I try to stay close to my higher power and to let that power manage my life. I use all the tools of my program today, and let my higher power run the show.

I trust the process of recovery, and today I trust my higher power. I have no need to ponder or worry about my pain recovery as long as I follow the simple steps my program outlines so clearly for me. My higher power has never failed me as long as I've had faith and done the next right thing in my recovery.

FEELINGS
EMOTIONAL BALANCE

....

"Research shows that the actual event is not the
cause of emotional pain, but the way the person
experiences and reacts to the event results in a pattern
of recurrent responses; e.g., fear, anxiety, and anger
are expressed as a headache."
A Day without Pain

Everyone in this world has suffered—I am not unique in that
regard, although in my active addiction I often felt that my suffering
was so much greater than that of other people that it entitled me to
behave with impunity—until the day came when I woke up
and entered recovery.

Today I don't berate myself for feeling pain over life's painful
events, and I don't prolong the agony of them by refusing to feel
my pain when it is fresh, or by buffering the pain with substances
or behaviors as I did in the past. Today I can identify my painful
feelings and process them as they occur, so that I don't express them
inappropriately. I stay in recovery, and I allow myself to feel all
of my feelings, the good and the bad.

*Feelings come and go; feelings cannot harm me unless I dwell in them
and use them as an excuse to avoid the work of recovery.*

ACCEPTANCE

PHYSICAL BALANCE

"Whatever positive changes you want to make in your
life, acceptance of how and where you are at the
present moment is one of the keys to moving forward."
Pain Recovery: How to Find Balance and
Reduce Suffering from Chronic Pain

Some days are better than others. I may feel healthy and
empowered one day, and the next feel like nothing has changed for
the better. As far as my physical balance is concerned, many times
absolutely nothing has changed except my perception. On days like
this I accept the physical limitations I may have, but I also realize
what I can do and concentrate on those things.

Regardless of how I'm feeling on a given day, I accept my physical
health without resistance. This is what it means to be in recovery.
Otherwise, I simply make matters worse. There is no standing still
in recovery. Either I'm moving forward and progressing in my
recovery, or I'm moving backward into a relapse. I can't afford to
fight my physical health on any given today.

*Regardless of how I am feeling, I am in acceptance of my physical
health. I am friends with my body, my pain, and also the parts of me
that are healthy and strong. All parts of me are in this together.*

THOUGHT PROCESS

MENTAL BALANCE

....

"Frustration and anger lead to increased muscle tension and
stress, which generally lead to increased sensations of pain."
Pain Recovery: How to Find Balance and
Reduce Suffering from Chronic Pain

One of my tasks in ongoing daily pain recovery is to monitor and
intervene on my negative thought processes right away, especially
on days when I'm in pain. If I'm frustrated because the breakfast
toast gets burned, I don't allow myself to think, "I hate mornings,"
"That toaster never worked right," or "What a lousy day this is
turning out to be." I realize that sometimes the toast gets burned,
and that's okay; maybe the eggs will be better.

That's a frivolous example, but it illustrates the way my thinking can
quickly turn negative—and the correlation between my negative
thoughts and beliefs and my level of pain can quickly become a
vicious cycle. My thoughts can spiral downward as they trigger my
pain, and my pain can trigger more negative thoughts. Negative
thoughts can easily translate into my own suffering, muscle tension,
and stress and amplify pain signals, triggering more of them. The
longer a cycle continues without an intervention in my thinking,
the more out of balance I become.

*When I feel pain, anger, or frustration, I focus on ignoring my negative
thoughts and increasing my positive self-talk to decrease my feelings of
frustration, anger, depression, hopelessness, and helplessness, knowing
that positive thoughts and feelings lower stress and tension and
decrease my pain in a way that medication never could.*

DRAMA
EMOTIONAL BALANCE

"Where there are no tigers,
a wildcat becomes self-important."
Korean proverb

I know that conflict and disappointment are natural parts of life, but sometimes it seems that these little annoyances can trigger my emotions to the point that I explode in anger or tears. I've even been called a "drama queen" or "drama king," terms I know are not flattering and that usually refer to a person with a demanding or overbearing personality who tends to overreact to seemingly minor incidents. Someone who seems to think they are too important for life's little difficulties—*that's* not me. Or is it?

I have to admit that sometimes it is. Before I entered recovery, my medications softened the effects of everyday annoyances; as long as I had my meds, little things didn't bother me. Today, although I've learned to live with chronic pain without abusing medication, my temper is ready to flare at times. But living a program of recovery, working toward humility, and understanding that I am not the center of the universe help me react sanely and compassionately to life's little stresses.

I relax and take it easy today, knowing that all my needs are provided for as long as I stay close to my higher power by working my program of recovery. I don't need to "sweat the small stuff." I can enjoy life, even when things don't go exactly the way I want them to. I don't need to rage or cry. I can remain calm and serene in my recovery.

CONTROL

SPIRITUAL BALANCE

....

*"Suffering is what you are feeling when
you're angry because it hurts; when you get
depressed because the pain won't stop."*
A Day without Pain

My suffering comes from something inside me that is still holding on, still trying to control my pain and to control my reaction to it, and this affects my spiritual balance. Being out of balance in any way can lead to suffering. Suffering is not something that I have to live with today, because I have a spiritual connection with a power that can help me deal with the pain instead of trying to control it.

When I accept that my pain is beyond my control, like almost everything else, I realize it's not something that I need to try to manage any longer. "Pain management" did not work for me, and only led to my becoming addicted to the pain medication.

I surrender today; I relinquish control, accept, do the footwork, work my pain recovery program, and find peace with my pain, and in doing so I find freedom from suffering.

*I do not hold onto the illusion of control; instead I focus
on what I can do to promote my recovery rather than what I
cannot do about my pain.*

EXPECTATIONS

RELATIONSHIPS

*"Give thanks for unknown blessings
already on their way."*
Native American proverb

What I expect often happens; however, sometimes, despite my efforts, things don't quite live up to my expectations, hopes, and desires, and then I become resentful. I can become bitter, and start thinking that things will never work out the way I want them to. I can forget how much better my life became when I entered recovery and stopped trying to manage it all on my own.

I learn the difference between my wants and my needs, between having expectations that are bound to create resentments when they are unmet and having confidence that my needs will be met when I work my program of recovery. Unexpected blessings are on their way—this I believe.

I expect the process of recovery to work for me. I expect prayer, meditation, meetings, steps, sponsorship, counseling, therapy, and living pain-medication-free to work for me and to ease my pain. And that's an expectation I can count on; the process does work— if I work it.

JUNE

19

NONJUDGMENTAL
PHYSICAL BALANCE

....

"Accepting others as they are does not mean we
must endure unacceptable judgments or actions
from them. It means, without anger or retaliation,
we acknowledge our powerlessness over the
judgments and actions of others. When we make this
acknowledgment, we find it easier to accept ourselves
even with our imperfections. In turn, when we accept
ourselves as whole and adequate, we are more able to
enjoy relations with others and accept their humanness
and imperfections. Another gift of acceptance is when
we are able to accept ourselves, we find the judgment
of others often loses its sting."
Of Character: Building Assets in Recovery

Other people don't have the power to hurt me. They only have the
power I give them. Their judgments of me only carry the weight
that I give them. Maybe the person judging me is actually doing
me a favor by shining a light on something about myself I need to
change. Whatever the case, the judgments of others do not have
power to hurt me unless I allow them to.

*The judgments of others toward me are not my problem. If I'm judging
something I dislike in someone else, then I need to work on myself
instead of concentrating on what's "wrong" with them. I work on me,
allowing others the right to do the same for themselves. Their opinion
of me is none of my business.*

FORGIVENESS
MENTAL BALANCE

"Let us forgive each other. Only then will we live in peace."
Leo Nikolaevich Tolstoy

My frustration, anger, and resentment toward medical professionals only compounded my pain and suffering. By masking my hurt and hopelessness with these negative emotions, I found temporary distraction from my pain through blame. When these emotions gave way to self-pity, I settled into the role of a victim, sometimes becoming terribly depressed. This threatened to make my pain worse.

I've found that letting go of resentment toward my doctors and other medical professionals was a good step in liberating me from the emotional bondage that magnifies my pain. Although I have many justifiable, logical, negative thoughts and feelings, giving in to thinking about them only makes me a victim again and keeps me in the cycle of perpetual unhappiness. I forgive the medical professionals who treated me; they were only trying to help. Perhaps they had never learned the techniques I now know to reduce my pain without resorting to medications—doctors don't know everything, after all.

I can also take responsibility for my part—after all, in the past I was all too willing to manipulate doctors to acquire the medication I craved. Today I know that medication is not the answer; I use my program of recovery to enable me to let go of my more difficult feelings.

Through forgiveness toward others and acceptance of my part in the past management of my pain, I work toward a future in pain recovery. Forgiveness feels much better than anger and resentment.

MODERATION, NOT EXTREMES

EMOTIONAL BALANCE

....

"Just paying attention to what we are feeling changes
the feeling. Being willing to acknowledge and accept
your limitations and feel them as they arise may help
remove their negative power."

A Day without Pain

Gut-wrenching despair and lighthearted exhilaration—I've known
both extremes. My emotions seem to exist not in the middle of the
spectrum, but at the extreme outward edges. Living in emotional
extremes is exhausting—especially when I'm in pain. The added
stress of feeling super-sad, or even super-elated, takes a toll on me
and makes me feel that perhaps I'm just too sensitive for this world.

Of course, that's not true; I'm here, in this world, therefore I belong
here. And I have everything I need in my program of recovery to
help me live, grow, and thrive here. I just have to breathe, calm
myself, and remind myself that nothing is either as bad or as good
as it seems and that I have tools and abilities I can call on to help
myself. (And I also remember that nothing—good or bad—lasts
forever.) Feelings of despair will vanish eventually, to be replaced
by feelings of elation. My job is to find the balance between the
extremes; that is where recovery lives.

I am aware of my tendency to be in emotional extremes, especially
in recovery, when my feelings, all of them, are often more magnified
because they are not being masked by medication. I feel better today,
which means that I have an increased capacity to feel my feelings more
deeply and intensely.

RECOVERY WORKS

SPIRITUAL BALANCE

"Only recently have researchers found that chronic
pain itself changes the brain in ways that scientists
have yet to fully understand. They believe, however,
that chronic pain causes many of the emotions that
are also associated with addiction, such as fear, anxiety,
depression, and unhappiness. This finding muddies
an already murky picture."

A Day without Pain

The Twelve Steps have been said to be a "simple solution for
complicated people." While the background, facts, research, causes,
solutions, cures, treatments, and effects of chronic pain may be
up for debate, one simple fact rings true: The Twelve Steps are a
solution. I can rest easier knowing that while the debate continues
about the nature of my disease, the nature of recovery is clear.

I work with my sponsor and support system; I pray and meditate;
I attend meetings, and don't abuse medication; and I feel better.
Doctors can worry about the nature of and cure for chronic
pain and addiction; I can focus on living. I don't need a team of
researchers to tell me what I've already experienced firsthand:
Chronic pain in recovery feels much better than chronic pain in
addiction. Of that much I am sure.

*While there is fear and uncertainty about the exact nature of some of
my ailments, I practice faith today by investing in one thing I don't
need a science experiment to prove works: recovery.*

SPIRITUAL AWAKENING

RELATIONSHIPS

....

"The secret of health for both mind and body
is not to mourn for the past, worry about the future,
or anticipate troubles, but to live in the present
moment wisely and earnestly."
Siddhartha Gautama, the Buddha

It is easy for me to forget that what I've learned in recovery to
deal with my chronic pain will also help me when I am dealing
with other people, places, or events in my own life that cause
me emotional pain. But the same principles hold true for all
pain, physical or emotional: If I feed a relationship problem
with sorrow over the past or anxiety over the future, the problem
becomes worse, just as my chronic pain becomes worse the more
I mourn my past health or worry about my future condition. But
if I remember to stay in the moment, to breathe and practice
the principles and tools I have learned in recovery, then my
relationships heal just as my chronic pain heals, and become easier
to bear. My spirituality awakens when I stay in the present.

Pain, physical or emotional, may not go away completely. But I
know today that I can cope with things that I didn't think I possibly
could before, by staying in the present moment.

*I use the tools I've learned in my program of recovery, particularly
prayer and meditation, to keep me in the "now." That is where my
higher power is, and where I am safe and free, and where my spirit
is awake. What a beautiful feeling!*

DEALING WITH CRAVING
PHYSICAL BALANCE

....

"Craving is a normal part of the process of drug
dependence and recovery. Wanting relief from
pain makes sense, but pain recovery consists
of dealing with pain differently."
Pain Recovery: How to Find Balance and
Reduce Suffering from Chronic Pain

I remind myself today that if I do not put drugs, including
the drug alcohol, into my body, the chance of having a true
"craving" is almost nil. Thoughts of using come and go, but
I must honestly admit that a mere thought is not a craving.
I am not bound to give in to it.

Thoughts of using are almost natural for someone like me, who
was once addicted to medication. My problem really arises when I
start to beat myself up for that thought and think there's something
wrong with my recovery. There is nothing wrong with my recovery
when I think about using medication or drugs; it's natural for me
to "go there" because of my former dependence. But I simply
remember and remind that voice that tells me using would be the
answer that in spite of whatever pain I'm feeling today, it's still
better than the damage and destruction that I caused to my body
and to those around me when I was using medication or other
substances to manage my pain.

*If I find that I'm thinking about using drugs, instead of feeling
ashamed I focus on the tools of recovery my program has given me—
meetings, service, sponsorship, prayer, and meditation.*

SPIRITUALITY

MENTAL BALANCE

"Every natural fact is a symbol of some spiritual fact."
Ralph Waldo Emerson

Even when I'm unsure of my path, there is a higher power that guides me. The voice of that power is subtle, soft, and internal; it's an inner knowingness that takes time and effort to hear, listen to, and trust. For me, spirituality is conversation with that voice.

In my life, I have faced, and continue to face, illness, pain, and disease—I'm human. My mind may wander when this happens. The voice in my head asks, "Why me, why is this happening to me?" Spirituality moves my mind toward understanding and accepting my pain, illness, or disease. Of course, it's hard to understand and accept pain and illness when I can't get it under control. That's when I need to listen to the voice that says, "It's okay; I will get through this, and I do not need to abuse medication."

In recovery, acceptance is vital. I accept my pain; I also accept the voice of spirituality that is within me. When I choose to fight pain, illness, or disease, when I engage in the conversation of the mind that reverts to self-pity, doubt, shame, and guilt, I do not make space for the whisper of spirituality that is the key to making any physical progress.

The whisper of spirituality gets louder the less I engage in the conversation with the disease. I choose surrender and acceptance. I accept my body, its chronic pain, illnesses, and limitations, knowing I cannot change my circumstances but that I can choose to accept my condition. I work each day to improve my life.

FEEDING THE WOLF I WANT TO WIN

EMOTIONAL BALANCE

> "If you care enough for a result,
> you will most certainly attain it."
> William James

I am reminded of a story I learned about in the book *Pain Recovery,* about two wolves. I remember the stories I hear from others in recovery and think about how they apply to my life today. Every day I stay in recovery, I learn more, and I know today that the results I care about are the results I work to attain.

A Cherokee elder was teaching his grandchildren about life. He said to them, "A fight is going on inside me…It is a terrible fight between two wolves. One wolf represents fear, anger, envy, sorrow, regret, greed, arrogance, self-pity, guilt, resentment, inferiority, lies, false pride, and superiority. The other stands for joy, peace, love, hope, sharing, serenity, humility, kindness, benevolence, friendship, empathy, generosity, truth, compassion, and faith. This same fight is going on inside you, and inside every other person too."

The children considered what their grandfather had said. "Which wolf will win?" They asked.

The old Cherokee simply replied, "The one you feed."
—*Author unknown*

There are two wolves inside me, too. I feed the one that I want to win, knowing that both are there, and either is capable of winning on any given day, depending on which is stronger.

BELIEF/HIGHER POWER

SPIRITUAL BALANCE

"Spirituality helps me reconnect with that which is greater than me and helps me connect with a higher purpose. Spirituality broadens my horizons by lifting me out of narrow, self-centered focus and helps me find meaning in my difficulties. If I think of pain or addiction as an affliction or a curse; if I think of myself as a victim; if my mind frame is one of self-pity, my capacity to experience relief from chronic pain and stay clean is greatly diminished."

Adapted from Pain Recovery: How to Find Balance and Reduce Suffering from Chronic Pain

I may not always "feel" spiritual or "holy," but I must always be aware that there is a power greater than myself that is loving and benevolent, and that will work in my life if I do the next right thing and remain humble and teachable. My pain may be great, but my higher power is greater.

Spiritual beliefs are personal and individual, but as I come to believe in a power greater than myself and strengthen that belief in recovery, I continue to remember that my higher power is loving, caring, and non-judgmental, and only wants what is best for me.

TRUST AND FEEDBACK

RELATIONSHIPS

....

"Sometimes trust is a matter of giving someone the
benefit of the doubt. Other times trust requires us to
step into the unknown and try something outside our
comfort zone. The trust is not just what we do; it is the
attitude and intention with which we do it."
Of Character: Building Assets in Recovery

Saying that I trust in someone, whether in another person
important to my recovery or in my higher power, is easy. Living
as if I trust him or her is more difficult. I might say I trust that the
circus performer will be able to push the wheelbarrow across the
high wire—that's easy; truly trusting him to do so would give me
the confidence to get into the wheelbarrow and let him push
me across the wire as well!

In recovery, I've experienced the way my higher power works for
my benefit and that of others in my fellowship. I grow to trust my
higher power and to trust in the process of recovery. I allow myself
to follow suggestions today, suggestions that might not have made
sense to me before, but I trust that the people in my life today with
whom I've surrounded myself only want what's good for me. I trust
that my higher power only wants what's good for me. And I know
that I only want what's good for me today.

*Today I take suggestions and follow directions, and trust that the
results will be for my continued growth and happiness.*

PLANNING, POSITIVE ACTION

PHYSICAL BALANCE

"Unless commitment is made, there are only
promises and hopes, but no plans."
Peter F. Drucker

As long as I remember that I am in the footwork business, and that
my higher power is in the results business, I can plan for and do
what I know is right, then leave the results up to my higher power.

I take positive action today for my recovery. My planning consists
of knowing what to do that will keep my recovery strong. I already
know what meetings I will attend this week, I have accumulated
phone numbers from other members of my recovery fellowship, and
I have recovery literature on hand. I have set aside time each day
for prayer and meditation. I have a commitment in my fellowship
that I make time to complete. This is the kind of planning I do
today. I don't stress over the minutiae regarding upcoming events,
but I do have a plan of recovery today.

*Recovery is a lifelong process, a process of working toward goals—
perhaps never achieving them, but doing the work just the same.
I will remember that recovery is a fluid and ever-changing process,
and to be good to myself and make gentle, incremental changes—
course corrections—when needed.*

PRAYER

MENTAL BALANCE

....

*"Learn and practice prayer and meditation.
Ask your higher power daily to guide you according
to His or Her will. Believe that 'if God brings you to it,
He will bring you through it.'"*
The Soul Workout: Getting and Staying Spiritually Fit

Pain and fear travel together, and whether one causes the other doesn't really matter to me anymore; I'm no longer ruled by fear or pain. Instead, today I have many resources that can reduce my pain and the accompanying fear, and chief among them is prayer.

I ask for strength and courage in my daily prayers, and they come— strength to withstand my pain and courage to allay my fear.

Using prayer, I no longer cut myself short of life-enhancing experience. Overcoming fear of pain has been possible through prayer. Ongoing, continuous prayer is a necessity in a successful pain recovery program. Sometimes this may be in quiet, structured times, and other times it's a silent thought process that happens while in the middle of a large group of people, while exercising, while sitting in a meeting. Using prayer to walk through fear teaches me what I'm capable of—and it's usually much more than I had ever thought.

I focus my mind on prayer rather than pain, rather than fear. Pain and fear exist; they are part of the human condition, and therefore part of my condition. However, I no longer need to linger in either state—I can cut both of them down to manageable size through the power of prayer.

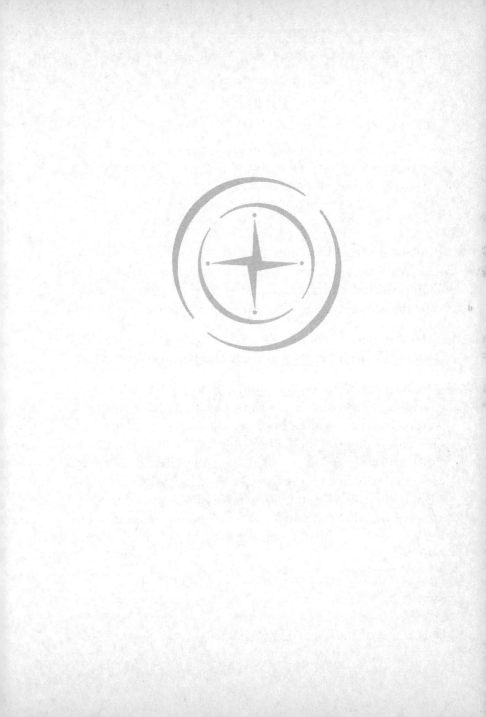

{ JULY }

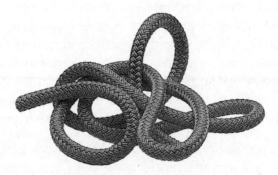

SELF-IMAGE

EMOTIONAL BALANCE

....

"A jug fills drop by drop."
Siddhartha Gautama, the Buddha

Building my self-esteem and my self-image takes time. Little by little, as I perform "esteemable acts," I grow in self-esteem, and my self-image improves bit by bit. I wish it could happen overnight, but it is a process. Like everything else worth having in my life, building my self-image takes time, but it can be done, and I'm doing it.

I'm doing it by being responsible and self-supporting, helping others, living in acceptance, working the steps of my recovery program. Improved self-esteem in turn improves my self-image. I see that I am in fact a capable person to whom others look for help. I see that I am a contributing member of my household, my fellowship, and my community. I begin to hold my head up high, something I may not have done in my active addiction to pain medication. I no longer need feel shame and guilt. I know that I am as good as anyone else — no better, and certainly no worse. Today, I'm happy to be "good enough," and my self-image benefits from that happiness.

My improved self-image means that today I take care of my personal hygiene and my living space to the best of my ability. I take pride in the appearance I present to the world. This is not egotism or vanity; it is the healthy expression of a good self-image.

I make sure I'm taking care of my self-image, both internally and externally, by taking care of myself with good hygiene, cleanliness, and personal internal development through my program of recovery.

WILLINGNESS
SPIRITUAL BALANCE

....

"When we are unwilling to consider we could be wrong
or when a 'position' is so sacred it feels heretical to
question it, we place ourselves on dangerous ground."
Of Character: Building Assets in Recovery

I talk to someone in my support group. I hear something at a
meeting or read something in my recovery literature. I feel an
intense reaction to it. Pain recovery encourages me to lean into the
conversation or information rather than away from it. I practice
willingness to achieve spiritual balance by seeking to understand, to
hear, to listen, and to internalize what is being said, especially when
I don't agree with it. I put one foot in front of the other and practice
the principle of Step Three in the Twelve Steps—turning my will
and life over to a higher power. Through the practical application
of willingness, I shift my own consciousness, understanding, and
feelings. I find spiritual balance. I integrate my own understanding
of life into that of the world around me.

*I actively work to be part of the world around me rather than apart
from that world. Willingness is my connection to freedom and a daily
reprieve from the intensity of chronic pain in isolation.*

THE NATURE OF BALANCE

RELATIONSHIPS

"Balance is not static, but a fluid state, in more-or-less constant flux, much like the ebb and flow of the waves of the ocean. As the circumstances of my life change, so will my state of balance. Balance is the journey, not the destination, and I'm the navigator. No one else steers my ship, but people, circumstances, and events can create obstacles along the way. Along my journey, the wind can be an obstacle, either blowing me off-course, or it can be a tool I can harness to move myself in the right direction."

Pain Recovery: How to Find Balance and
Reduce Suffering from Chronic Pain

It's tempting to wish that balance in relationships, once achieved, will remain firmly set, now and forever. However, think of a seesaw, or of a scale. The seesaw teeters but can be brought into balance, and the arms of the scale can, too, but this requires constant attention—a little more weight here, a little less there. For my relationships to maintain balance in recovery, I must be attentive to their shifting, ongoing, changing needs, and make adjustments as required.

I navigate the seas of life and recovery, knowing that I need to make adjustments as I move along, responding, not reacting, to situations in life, and focusing on the excitement of the journey, learning every day more about the waters I travel.

POWERLESSNESS

PHYSICAL BALANCE

"A team of American researchers at Brown University
in Rhode Island showed that even a single dose of
morphine physically changed the brain, and the
change persisted long after the effects of the drug had
worn off. Other studies have shown that a single dose of
methamphetamine has resulted in brain damage."

A Day without Pain

Since I've used drugs, my brain has changed. I'm powerless over
that fact. I'm different from the person I was before using pain
medication. But I've got the power to rewire my brain, even though
it will always be altered as a result of drug use. I remember this as
I move forward through my recovery, especially when I find myself
comparing myself to others and thinking things that hurt me in
the long run, like: Why can others take pain medication without
becoming addicted? Why do I have to be different? Ultimately,
it doesn't matter why—what matters is that today I know I'm
powerless over the initial thoughts and feelings that continue to
separate me from others. This is the downward spiral that leads back
to addictive, acting-out behavior and eventually active addiction. I
have power over my second thoughts, my actions, and my recovery.

*I recognize I'm powerless over my addiction, chronic pain, and the
results of those two things, such as the changes to my brain caused by
past drug use, and in surrendering to this recognition, I find the power
to rewire my brain and reprogram myself with my recovery program.*

RELAPSE PREVENTION, POSITIVE ACTION

MENTAL BALANCE

"I understand that the four points of balance—physical, emotional, mental, spiritual—are the essence of who I am. My state of balance is directly related to my actions and behaviors.

If I'm not actively practicing the principles of pain recovery I will relapse—not just on opioids but on unhealthy behaviors that only make my pain worse. If I relapse, I'll lose sight of the advantages of recovery and seek out short-term, immediate gratification.

To be in pain recovery means staying in balance, and that includes my full acceptance of the problem and fully implementing the solution in all areas of my life. When I have found balance in body, mind, emotion, and spirit, relapse prevention is better labeled recovery maintenance and enhancement. Pain recovery maintenance, relapse prevention means continuously monitoring the four points of balance."

Adapted from Pain Recovery: How to Find Balance and Reduce Suffering from Chronic Pain

Imbalance usually results from not practicing what I've learned in pain recovery. I need to be careful not to judge myself for letting up on my recovery, but just correct the imbalances and stay consistent. I recognize the signs of relapse and learn how to take corrective action as early as possible. I take action to correct, get back in balance, and resume recovery.

I stay close to others in my pain recovery support group—these people remind me to practice the tools of pain recovery in order to stay in balance.

ANXIETY

EMOTIONAL BALANCE

··

"Every tomorrow has two handles. We can take hold of
it with the handle of anxiety or the handle of faith."
Henry Ward Beecher

Anxiety is a form of fear. It's a feeling I get when I'm afraid of the
way something is going to turn out. It's the fear of how I'll handle
something that hasn't happened yet. It's the discomfort I feel when
I'm doing something new or different. I sometimes get anxious
before I get out of bed in the morning, and the feeling follows me
wherever I go. There isn't a cure *per se* for my anxiety, but I've
learned techniques that can help.

First and foremost is not letting it get me out of balance and not letting
the fear get "off the charts." Once that happens, I may start reacting
and making decisions from that feeling. When I'm feeling anxious
I acknowledge it to another person, write about it, or do something
active to get the anxiety out of my body. Movement, working out,
walking, yoga; these activities burn off the energy generated by anxiety,
and the feelings that go along with it often subside.

Under my anxiety is fear that somehow my needs aren't going to
get met, that I'm going to suffer, be neglected, not get what I want
or need. When I remember that my higher power meets all my
needs, if not my wants, I can handle the fear without having the
anxiety that is usually attached.

I face my fear, and turn it over to my higher power. Sometimes I do
this a minute at a time. If I don't have faith enough for this, then
I ask for faith until it comes.

AWAKENING

SPIRITUAL BALANCE

"I close my eyes in order to see."
Paul Gauguin

I was probably the last one among my family and close friends to know that I had a problem with pain medication, that my behavior was out of line, or that I needed help. My spiritual awakening was not like the "burning bush" of Scripture—at first, it was simply realizing what those around me had long known.

The spiritual awakening I receive as a result of pain recovery also encompasses the realization that my higher power has always been there and is not something I need to go outside myself to find. My spirituality has always been inside of me, but when it was clouded by diseased thinking and abuse of medication, I was not aware of or receptive to that spark of life that was (and is) already within me. When I entered recovery, I learned to become still, to open myself up, and to awaken to the light within.

The spiritual awakening may in fact be of the "burning bush" variety, but odds are that what is alight within me is the spirit and heart that is inside me, which I've been too numb to feel, and which others may have watched burning for much longer than I've ever realized.

What serenity there is in knowing I have the light of recovery inside me, and can tap into its warmth and brilliance whenever I need to.

SEX AND SEXUALITY

RELATIONSHIPS

"If you want to be loved, be lovable."
Ovid

Although chronic pain can challenge my ability to enjoy a healthy and satisfying sex life, I remind myself that sexual intimacy doesn't have to "measure up" to any standards other than my own and that of my partner. Sex is an important part of my life and my relationships, so it's worth the extra effort that is sometimes required to have a healthy sex life in pain recovery.

I am aware that good sex starts with communication, and so I communicate with my partner about my needs and desires, feelings and insecurities. I communicate my love and commitment. And I give and receive pleasure to the best of my ability on any given day.

I remain open to new ways of expressing myself sexually, and don't judge myself or my partner for any perceived inability or lack. I welcome the opportunity to explore new ways to give and receive pleasure. I use my sexual powers for healing and joy, for myself and my partner. Today I believe this is the reason my higher power created us as sexual beings—to bring greater joy and happiness into each other's lives. I receive love as I give it to my partner today.

Chronic pain does not change my basic nature; like all human beings, I am sexual, and today I am free to enjoy my sexual nature in any way that does not harm, manipulate, or use others. Even if I can no longer enjoy activities that once brought me pleasure, I can appreciate the opportunity to expand my horizons sexually in my recovery.

IMPATIENCE/PATIENCE

PHYSICAL BALANCE

....

"Since chronic pain has no single cause or enabling
feature, treatment methods are extremely varied....
If something works once, it will work again if you keep
at it. Practice will enhance the benefits."

A Day without Pain

It's the nature of an addict to look for the quick fix. Even though
I'm in recovery, I really want the very first yoga, meditation,
acupuncture, or therapy session or recovery meeting I attend to
result in immediate relief. What I must remember is that recovery
is a process, and that I need to be patient in order to get the results I
want. I need to remember that I didn't necessarily become addicted
overnight—my chronic pain got progressively worse over a period
of time, and the recovery process takes time as well. Each day I
make a habit of doing something good for myself. It builds on the
previous day, expands on prior successes, until over time I realize
that I'm feeling better, have more flexibility, and have a greater
capacity for activity—I can sit and meditate longer, get into more
postures in yoga, handle deeper acupuncture, etc. I have built
good habits that produce good results in my recovery.

*I'm patient with the process of recovery, focusing on the habits
I'm forming today that will save my life tomorrow.*

PERFECTIONISM

MENTAL BALANCE

....

"The further I travel on the path of recovery,
the more I am able to accept myself
as a perfectly imperfect human."
Tails of Recovery: Addicts and the Pets That Love Them

Perfectionism is striving after what is unattainable, and therefore it's unrealistic. It's something I can use to justify doing nothing to move my recovery forward. If the very idea that I might not be able to do a thing perfectly prevents me from doing it at all, I have to look at that—am I being a perfectionist, or am I really being fearful? Lazy? Insecure? Do I have reservations that will sabotage my recovery if they are not overcome? Looking at my motives helps me realize that what I justify as "perfectionism" (which, after all, sounds socially acceptable) may in fact be something much less acceptable that I'd prefer not to look at.

Today I'll appreciate myself and my very real abilities, and remember that I am good enough for the task of recovery; that "I can do it." Rather than stagnating in a false "perfectionism," I'll take the steps needed in my recovery, whether I do them perfectly or not. After all, the only imperfect way to work on my recovery is to do nothing at all.

MEMORY
EMOTIONAL BALANCE

....

"All that we are is the result of what we have thought.
The mind is everything. What we think, we become."
Siddhartha Gautama, the Buddha

Memories of painful events might be buried deep in my unconscious mind, but that doesn't mean they are gone without a trace. The fact that the memory is buried means the sight, sound, smell, taste, or feeling that can trigger that memory is also buried. And because both the trigger and the memory are buried, I can end up depressed, fearful, angry, or upset without quite knowing why.

I may never fully "work through" my childhood or other past issues, although I try. They are part of what makes me who I am today, but I'm not a victim of them, nor do I need to be a perpetrator because of them. I actively work on these issues, with a therapist as well as with my sponsor, especially if they "come up" repeatedly. The last thing I want is to cause others pain because of my own unresolved issues. If I'm actively working a program of recovery, it usually doesn't take so long to realize I need to pause and realign my behavior with program principles to avoid hurting myself or others; that's the last thing I want to do today.

As part of my pain recovery program, I am committed to acknowledge and resolve my past issues, to ensure they are not intruding on my life today. This is part of "cleaning up my side of the street."

RESPONSIBILITY

SPIRITUAL BALANCE

....

"To be responsible we must know who we are and what
we are doing, as well as where we fit in the world."
Of Character: Building Assets in Recovery

Meetings, steps, sponsorship, friendship, and family give
me a sense of where I fit in the world today. While other activities,
like work, may be of importance to me, the truth is that when I was
suffering from chronic pain, abusing medication, and behaving in
an addictive, defective manner toward those in my life, nothing else
mattered. When I came to recovery, it was because nothing else
worked. Recovery becomes first in my life so that I can have success
in the other areas of my life that are important. My place
in the world is in recovery.

I make my place in the world my personal pain recovery program,
understanding that while everything else in my life is important, the
most important thing is my recovery, because without that I will not
have anything else to worry about or to enjoy!

SPIRITUALITY

RELATIONSHIPS

....

"Our intellect, emotions, thoughts, actions,
and relationships join together to form the essence
and expression of our spirit. Our spirit is the product
of all the parts of our life."
Of Character: Building Assets in Recovery

My spirit is not a thing apart from myself; my spirit is intricately and
intimately woven throughout all of me. It is in my consciousness,
my unconsciousness, my thoughts, and my actions. My spirit
connects me to you, and to my higher power. Knowing this, I am
careful always to strive to express only the highest and best of me,
aware that as I do, I am living in the world of the spirit as well as
the world of the flesh. My flesh is sometimes weak, or in pain.
However, my spirit is the part of me that withstands and transcends
my pain, and makes my life worth living.

*Spirituality to me means feeling all of my feelings, experiencing
all of my body, mind, and spirit. It's the integration of and
relationship among all four points of balance that make a whole
person. Knowing myself to be a spiritual being is having an ongoing
realization that there is a part of me that is connected to that
which always was and always will be.*

PEACE AND MEDITATION

PHYSICAL BALANCE

···

"Meditation is one of the most popular of alternative methods of pain relief. Practitioners say that when people meditate, they can increase the amount of natural painkillers in their body and stimulate the production of pleasurable chemicals. Meditation can encourage a sense of well-being, happiness, connectedness, and wholeness."

A Day without Pain

Meditation has its place as a daily practice in my life. Any peace I find without prayer and meditation is temporary, a fabricated peace that is held together with flimsy hopes and wish-filled dreams, not grounded in reality. These hopes and dreams tell me I can be instantly "fixed" by a person, place, or thing. But to really experience peace and connectedness in my body and mind, I need meditation. While there are many methods and teachers and techniques and traditions, the only wrong way to meditate is to not do it! However I meditate, skillfully or clumsily, I have confidence that if I meditate with the intention of improving my conscious contact with my higher power, and I do this regularly, I'll come to a point in my life where it becomes somewhat second nature to me. The addict in me will always seek a quick fix, and quick fixes are fleeting and temporary. The real "fix" provided by meditation takes time, but it lasts, and builds my recovery.

I am forming the habit of meditation as my preferred method of pain relief. Through meditation, I'm making a habit of encouraging my own well-being, being happy, connected, and whole.

POWER VS. VICTIM

MENTAL BALANCE

"I am, indeed, a king,
because I know how to rule myself."
Pietro Aretino

Rather than focusing on things I can no longer do, I attain mental balance by focusing my energy and thoughts on the things I *can* do. In doing so, I live in a power greater than my own, rather than being a victim of my chronic pain. I choose to do the things I can in my life. I set attainable goals and work toward them. I set forth to *do*. I take realistic pride in my accomplishments and share them with others, without bragging, but humbly. I am not the victim. I no longer suffer in silence. Adjusting my thinking this way, I can achieve mental balance—neither living in the faulty thinking that dwells only on what I can't do, nor living in grandiose dreams of achievements I can no longer realistically accomplish. I do what I can, appreciating what I can do when I rely on a power greater than myself, which is available to me when I work on my recovery.

When I am having thoughts of being a victim, I focus those thoughts instead on the ways in which I do have power today. I think first of what I can do, rather than what I cannot. I think first of what I will do, rather than what I did not or could not do because of my chronic pain.

PEACE

EMOTIONAL BALANCE

....

"I had found probably the one meeting,
the one place on earth that would allow me to relate
what I had done and not be judged for it.
At that meeting I knew somewhere deep in my soul
I had found a way to live with what I had done.
That day began my love affair with my twelve-step
fellowship and my journey of recovery."
Tails of Recovery: Addicts and the Pets That Love Them

I come to terms with my guilt and shame by sharing it with others
who have shared similar experiences. With them, I find more true
empathy, and I do not feel alone—more importantly, I see how my
experiences can help others. Guilt and shame in moderation can be
healthy feelings. They help frame my values and give me humility,
but in their extremes, they can be toxic. Through writing, sharing,
and listening, I'm freed from toxic shame and guilt that destroys,
and instead, I come to find peace with righteous and healthy guilt
and shame, turning it into a solution, a way of living in the
world with values and true humility.

*I write and journal about areas of my life over which I feel guilt and
shame. I do not feel guilt and shame for having guilt and shame,
because that is a natural part of life, but I no longer wallow in these
toxic emotions. I have a program that gives me the tools to clean up my
past and make right the wrongs I feel so guilty over. I move past guilt
and shame into recovery of body, mind, and spirit today.*

GROUNDED

RELATIONSHIPS

···

"The dialogue of searching almost always
results in our feeling more connected to the world
and to those to whom we listen."
Of Character: Building Assets in Recovery

Reaching out is often thought of as reaching out to people. But I
reach out to my higher power on a regular basis, as well. Often I
reach out to my higher power more than I do another person. My
higher power always has time for me—he's never on the phone,
at work, busy with friends or family, or sleeping! I reach out to my
higher power to achieve spiritual balance and connectedness. Over
time, as I achieve spiritual balance, I then reach out to others.
While during certain phases of recovery I need the fellowship
and support from other people, I take the most comfort in knowing
that my higher power is always there for me. I get connected
to that power first. All else follows.

*I reach out to my higher power regularly and consistently,
knowing that in building and strengthening that relationship,
my attempts to reach out to others will be all the more enhanced,
grounded, and spiritually balanced.*

VARIETY

PHYSICAL BALANCE

"There are a multitude of different techniques
and therapies to improve chronic pain and enhance
our lives. Most help physical pain, and some focus on
diminishing our suffering. Combining several modalities
makes the most sense, as each works differently;
using many different techniques allows me to
activate different body and mind systems, resulting
in positive outcomes: decreased pain and
suffering and improved function."

A Day without Pain

I do a little, try a little, see what works for me, and then practice
at those one or two things. I'm not expected, nor can I expect my
body, to be able to do it all—that's an addictive mind-set. Instead, I
form a habit of working a little bit from a variety of techniques for
pain relief into my routine. If I want to try something else, I start
out by doing it once. If it seems to work, then I can add it to my
"toolbox" of techniques. I take it easy, and add new activities one at
a time, discarding old practices that no longer work for me.

*I use multiple techniques and modalities to improve my pain. I
work a little, take a little from this-and-that, constantly refining and
improving, adjusting my routine to suit my needs and abilities.*

INTERVENING WITH HOPE

MENTAL BALANCE

"Where there's life, there's hope."
Terence

My physical pain is a reflection of my past and can overwhelm me in this present day and time. Rather than being overwhelmed, I can think about the progress I've made in pain recovery, and that gives me hope for the future.

I feel my pain mentally, physically, and/or emotionally, stemming from some situation or event that happened in the past. Because of this chronic pain, I'm reminded on a daily basis of that event. Sometimes this can be an ugly reminder of my past actions, or something that was completely beyond my control. Whatever the situation or event was, I do not have to live in the past. When I start to think about the past I intervene on that thought and replace it with a thought of hope for the future: a future filled with a life lived in pain recovery.

I accept that the pain I feel today is a reminder of the past—however, it does not have to rob me of the wonderful things the present and future hold.

SELF-AWARE VS. SELF-OBSESSED

EMOTIONAL BALANCE

·····

> "Oh, how great peace and quietness would
> he possess who should cut off all vain anxiety
> and place all his confidence in God."
> Thomas à Kempis

Nothing could be more annoying, to myself and to those close to me, than to become a person constantly taking my emotional pulse. Always asking myself, "How am I feeling right now?" is not a way to live. At the same time, it's important for me to be aware of my emotions in order to deal with them appropriately. Have I been walking around with anger and resentment? Am I sad today? Do I feel guilt or shame over something? What am I afraid of— and does someone in my support group know? Keeping feelings to myself will make my recovery stagnate. No matter how ugly or embarrassing they may be, sharing them is important.

I've learned that what I feel will get me loaded, but what I do will promote my recovery. Therefore, while I remain aware of my emotions, I don't let them deter me from doing the work of my recovery program. Whether I'm depressed, fearful, anxious, or excited, I still do the work of recovery. I attend and share at meetings, I talk to my sponsor, I read recovery literature, and I make sure I'm of service to others. These things take me out of morbid navel-gazing and improve my quality of life.

I'm aware of my feelings today, and take note of them; however, I do not let them deter me from doing the next right thing for my recovery.

HIGHER EMOTIONAL FUNCTIONING

SPIRITUAL BALANCE

"Spirituality can be defined as many things, but in essence it is that of functioning in the world with a heightened state of awareness of myself, my connection with a higher power, and a connectedness with those around me. This higher emotional functioning makes it possible for me to handle my feelings and the feelings of those I'm in contact with throughout the day. Spirituality can be thought of as the area of life concerned with matters of the spirit, beyond oneself, though not necessarily in the religious sense. Spirituality includes a sense of connection to something greater than myself, which may or may not include an emotional experience of religious awe or reverence. It also includes a sense of connection to others, including emotional intimacy and connection to the world around me—a feeling of belonging to a greater whole."

Adapted from Pain Recovery: How to Find Balance
and Reduce Suffering from Chronic Pain

While it may involve a religious practice of some kind or another, spirituality does not need to mean that I even believe in a particular higher power today. My spirituality, like recovery, is always changing and evolving. It means that I live a principle-centered life and believe in the inherent value of myself and of humankind.

The process of recovery allows me the freedom to choose what form my spirituality takes based on what is right for me. I reflect on what spirituality means for me today. I am grateful that pain recovery has given me the opportunity to choose the form my spirituality and its practice take.

CONNECTION TO OTHERS

RELATIONSHIPS

....

*"While we realize that chronic pain is
experienced differently by every individual,
we also must understand that those in chronic pain
are tied together in a unique association."*

A Day without Pain

When I was in my active addiction, the emotional pain of feeling alone, as if no one else understood the true depth of my suffering, was matched only by the physical sensations that seemed intolerable. Even with the use of medication, I could barely tolerate my physical chronic pain, because the effects of the medication over time actually just made the pain worse.

Finding freedom from pain medication has been a tremendous freedom, but the gift of having others who relate to and understand me has been icing on the cake from a higher power I had thought long ago abandoned me. I've found that higher power in the faces, voices, experiences, and strengths of others who have come before me and those who are following. I find strength in people who are in the process of recovery, and greater strength, which counteracts the emotional turmoil of my pain, in helping others. Disconnection to others was my bottom, while connection to others is my zenith.

I focus on my connection with others who are in pain recovery, knowing that the isolation of active addiction is offset only by the fellowship, community, caring, and sharing with others who are also on this path. Knowing this, I will never be alone again.

TYPES OF MEDITATION

PHYSICAL BALANCE

....

"Meditation quiets the chatter in our heads
and allows us to gain perspective."
Pain Recovery: How to Find Balance and
Reduce Suffering from Chronic Pain

There's only one wrong way to meditate, and that's to not meditate at all. There are many types of meditation, and many books and teachers I can use in order to try them. I try the ones that appeal to me first, then ask around to learn what other members of my fellowship practice. If what they do seems to work for them, then I may try their techniques as well. The important thing is that I try.

I don't become discouraged or criticize myself if I don't measure up to some imagined ideal of spiritual enlightenment. It's enough that I am making the effort to relax, to breathe, and to allow conscious contact with my higher power. That's what meditation means to me today.

I make a point of meditating, without judging myself harshly or comparing myself to others. When meditation becomes common practice, I remember the importance of the practice and honor the dedication I've made to myself.

COMMITMENT

MENTAL BALANCE

....

*"Commitment unlocks the doors of imagination,
allows vision, and gives us the 'right stuff'
to turn our dreams into reality."*
Unknown

The idea of commitment can be overwhelming—that is,
when we consider making a commitment that will cover a
long period of time. The whole idea of remaining opioid/pain
medication-free and active in pain recovery for the rest of my
life was overwhelming at first.

When I stop looking at my recovery as a lifelong commitment, it
becomes much easier to deal with. This is why the concepts of "just
for today" and "one day at a time" are important in recovery. I only
have to be clean and in pain recovery today. I can do anything for
one day that would be impossible to imagine doing for the rest of
my life. I know that if I renew my commitment to staying clean and
in pain recovery each day, then each day I will receive the
strength and guidance I need for that day's journey.

*Tomorrow's responsibilities and next week's bills can be left
for tomorrow, next week, next month, or next year. I stay focused on
what I can do today. What I cannot do today does not have a
hold on me the way it did before.*

POWERLESSNESS

EMOTIONAL BALANCE

....

"Give up the feeling of responsibility, let go your hold,
resign the care of your destiny to higher powers, be
genuinely indifferent as to what becomes of it all and
you will find not only that you gain a perfect inward
relief, but often also, in addition, the particular goods
you sincerely thought you were renouncing."

William James

Powerlessness is not helplessness. This is worth repeating and worth
remembering. Few things can make me feel more powerless than
my emotions, especially emotional extremes. Extreme emotion
may make me feel that I'm completely out of control. Whether
the extreme is elation or depression, when my emotions are out
of whack, the result is a fearsome feeling of lack of control that
reminds me of active addiction and unchecked chronic pain. I need
to take a breath, center myself through prayer and meditation,
and remember that "this, too, shall pass."

Once I can do this, I can remember that powerlessness is not
helplessness. I am not helpless today; today I have choices. I
can choose how to react to my seemingly out-of-control, out-of-
balance emotions. I can use the tools of recovery to recalibrate
my emotional responses to life on life's terms so that they don't
exacerbate my chronic pain or impede my recovery.

*I may be powerless over the addiction that I have; I may be powerless
over my chronic pain, but I do have power over my choices in life. My life
is not controlled by my chronic pain, and I have choices about the kind
of person I want to be today,*

PATIENCE

SPIRITUAL BALANCE

....

*"The two most powerful warriors
are patience and time."*
Leo Nikolaevich Tolstoy

Pain is intended to signify when something is wrong or "off" in my body. Chronic pain indicates a permanent dysfunction that is worrisome and wearisome. The most frustrating aspect of chronic pain is that it is rare to achieve sustained relief from it. In pain recovery, I work to ensure that my chronic pain, or the addiction associated with it, does not control my life. I take an active role in my recovery. I follow my doctor's advice, set realistic, manageable goals for myself, and keep a journal to find out what exacerbates my pain and what relieves it. I've learned that stress triggers an increase in pain. Tools such as deep breathing, meditation, and exercise/ movement are available to me today to reduce pain when I'm going through difficult times.

I am patient with myself, striving to understand that pain recovery takes time. While pain is my body's way of sending a message that something is wrong, through working toward spiritual balance I send a message back that I am okay today.

FOUR POINTS OF BALANCE

RELATIONSHIPS

"Emotions or feelings do not always occur in direct response to sensory events. Sometimes the events are internal like a headache or external like being stuck in traffic. It seems sometimes like it is the event that causes the emotion. I am reminded that it is actually my thought about such an event that triggers the emotion. How I think about the event, my beliefs, and how I interpret the event create my emotional responses. In turn, that emotional response has a lot of influence over my consequent action. Depending on my state of balance, I can respond to the exact same event differently under different circumstances. "

Adapted from Pain Recovery: How to Find Balance and Reduce Suffering from Chronic Pain

I remember that my chronic pain and the disease of addiction both color my perception today. Events may not mean exactly what I think they do, and it's a pretty good bet that the actions of others aren't intended to hurt me, although sometimes that's how I perceive them at the time.

I meditate on the day's events and think of how I could respond to the same event differently on a given day. Where I find myself reacting negatively, I make an effort to think of an alternative, positive way I want to react in the future. Where I find myself reacting positively, I note that as well, so that I can remember and use that information later.

POWER

PHYSICAL BALANCE

"I've learned that powerlessness is not helplessness.
I am certainly not helpless. I've been given everything
I need to make my way in this world. Accepting
powerlessness is accepting freedom; it allows the
weight of the world to fall from my shoulders. Accepting
my powerlessness goes hand-in-hand with trusting my
higher power to provide everything I need."

Adapted from The Soul Workout:
Getting and Staying Spiritually Fit

It doesn't feel like I have power over my chronic pain, and in many ways I *am* powerless. But I do have power over how I deal with, accept, and work through my life with chronic pain. Ironically, in expressing, or exerting, that power, I can actually decrease some level of the pain I'm in. This requires exerting power where I have it, and that is most notable in the physical habits I create for myself. On a daily, moment-by-moment basis, I must be focusing on my new habits. I can't expect that I'm going to create new habits for myself overnight or even over a year or two. It may take much longer, but that's why I have a higher power. I ask regularly for the power to carry out my higher power's will for me.

I have power in my life in creating my physical habits that accommodate and contribute to my pain recovery. I'm exerting power over those things I can and accepting powerlessness over the results.

WILLINGNESS

MENTAL BALANCE

"Even if strength fails, boldness at least
will deserve praise: In great endeavors even
to have had the will is enough."
Sextus Propertius

Willingness is a principle that is essential to pain recovery but does not come naturally to me. My ability to show up and participate in my recovery, even when I don't want to, is a huge asset in recovery. Being willing is a way to put open-mindedness into action. All that is required is that I be open-minded and able to try something new. Addiction and chronic pain are often parallel in that they force people into perpetual cycles of doing the same thing repeatedly. I started fearing any change, good or bad.

I never know what can help me until I try it for a while. I can have all the information in the world about a protocol, treatment, or process that may help me, but I'll forever be missing the crucial piece if I don't try it. One way I can renew my willingness for recovery is through surrendering old beliefs for a shot at something new.

By surrendering to my disease and admitting my powerlessness over it, I may find the willingness needed to continue in recovery, especially when that is difficult and painful and requires courage.

SUFFERING

EMOTIONAL BALANCE

....

"To suffering there is a limit; to fearing, none."
Sir Francis Bacon

Suffering is optional. I've learned in my recovery that I have two paths: either accepting my pain or trying to avoid it through the use of drugs. I choose the path of suffering when I attempt to eliminate all pain by avoiding, masking, and medicating. This approach does not eliminate all pain, and results in imbalance in other areas of my life. The more I attempt to avoid, mask, and medicate, the greater my suffering is. Today I choose the path to pain recovery, and the way I go about it is different. Some days it's exercise, walking, going to work, etc. That means I must give up the quest for "no more pain" and acknowledge and accept that some pain will likely always be with me. Recovery starts with recognizing that my pain is a part of my life and does not need to be feared or avoided. I lean into the pain by simply allowing it to be there without resistance.

I have become empowered to change the way I experience my pain.
I have changed my goals from "no more pain" to achieving
manageable levels of physical pain, increasing function, and reducing
suffering. I am not pain-free, but I am pain-less.

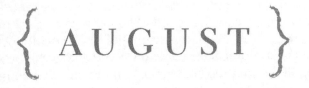

{ AUGUST }

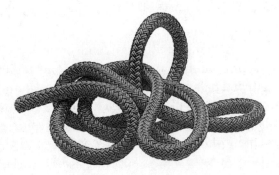

STRENGTH

SPIRITUAL BALANCE

"He who gains a victory over other men is strong,
but he who gains a victory over himself is all-powerful."
Lao Tzu

Emotional, mental, and spiritual strength increase my physical strength. When I'm having a difficult day from chronic pain, I find strength in my spiritual connection. Sometimes that connection may be the only defense holding me back from active addiction. Chronic pain makes it difficult for my mind to focus. The last thing I'm thinking of is being strong because I feel so weakened from the pain. I desire so deeply to live a normal life. Recovery has given me the ability to see more clearly, but some days I just can't reach the goal that I've set in recovery. During these times I reach into a place that is untouched, untainted, and untarnished by my chronic pain. This inner and higher self, this transcendent place, is protected from the physicality of my chronic pain and addiction.
I find strength and balance in all points of my program by calling on the spiritual part within me. Each part of my program is invigorated and charged: Mentally I focus on this spirit, emotionally I feel the memory of having once been connected, and physically my body at least eases a little, knowing that I'm not going to abandon it again to darkness, despair, and addiction.

When everything is out of balance, I call upon and focus on one of the four points of balance to help all the others to find their balance. Even though I may not feel as strong as I would like, I keep a strong spiritual program that helps me in all points of my recovery program.

1

UNPREDICTABLE NATURE OF PAIN

RELATIONSHIPS

....

"I need to remember that my pain is unpredictable and
this is a strain on more than just me. The people I live with,
who try to help and care for me, particularly on those
bad days, can be just as affected by my pain as I am.
I get to remember this and remember others around
me in my recovery today. When I'm having worse days,
the strain on those who love me, trying to cover more
responsibilities, is added to already existing conflict or
tension and their suffering can be quite profound.... By
recognizing the impact of my pain on those around me
and communicating clearly when I'm feeling better or
worse, without demanding attention or sympathy, I can
help ease the pressure on my loved ones."
Adapted from Pain Recovery: How to Find Balance
and Reduce Suffering from Chronic Pain

One day my pain may be quite subdued, making those who care
for me happy, as they mistake the temporary lessening of pain
for a permanent release. But the next day, pain may spike again,
disappointing me and my caregivers, unless we remember that my
chronic pain is unpredictable. By keeping our expectations
in check and practicing the principles of recovery, we show caring
and concern for each other.

*I don't overstate my case, but I don't leave those around me guessing
about whether or how much I'm in pain on any given day. I remember
there are times when their pain, though perhaps not physical, is as great
as my own, and I try to be sensitive to their needs as well as my own.*

GRIEF

MENTAL BALANCE

....

"Time is a physician that heals every grief."
Diphilus

My grief is no greater and no less than that felt by others. However, my chronic pain magnifies everything I experience. At times, I dramatize my grief, believing no one else has ever suffered the way I do. It would be easy to play the victim at times like this, falling back on old habits. However, in pain recovery, I've learned that I am not unique; I am not even alone. Others can help with their experience, strength, and hope. And I in turn can help others, instead of dwelling on my own pain.

I remember that my body and my mind have been provided with tools to help fade or lessen memories of painful experiences. These natural defense mechanisms exist to protect me from my past and to allow me to live in the present. When I'm feeling extreme mental or emotional pain, I keep my thoughts focused on what I need to do for my pain recovery and for my physical and spiritual well-being, knowing that doing so helps my body, emotions, and spirit to react with natural defenses, which every human possesses, to deal with such pain.

I accept and appreciate my ability to accept and heal from my painful past. Time heals all wounds—and during that time when I'm in grief and suffering from loss, during the time it takes to naturally heal, I think first of my physical recovery, my pain recovery.

EXPECTATIONS

MENTAL BALANCE

....

"The greatest loss of time is delay and expectation,
which depend upon the future. We let go the present,
which we have in our power, and look forward to
that which depends upon chance, and so relinquish
a certainty for an uncertainty."

Seneca

Expectations are particularly dangerous, in part because they are
so subtle that I may not recognize them for what they are. I may
have an expectation that pain can be completely removed from my
life, that after pain-free periods the pain will not return, or that after
actively participating in my recovery I will not revert back
to destructive behavior or negative thinking. I must remember
to try my best to live expectation-free, to allow life to unfold,
and to accept the will of my higher power, trusting that it will
always be for my ultimate good.

*I educate myself about pain recovery and addiction, to know that
it is human to err and to be imperfect. Chronic pain and addiction
are diseases that lie patiently and wait, and given the right set of
circumstances, they will invade my life again through expectations
and many other avenues.*

COPING WITH SUFFERING

EMOTIONAL BALANCE

....

"Pain is a part of life and cannot be avoided."
Pain Recovery: How to Find Balance and
Reduce Suffering from Chronic Pain

Pain is inevitable. I have accepted this and discovered the
things that I can do today despite pain. I understand that pain is
multidimensional. It's more than my body experiencing aching,
throbbing, stinging, burning, or whatever other sensations plague
me. It is enduring loss (emotional), feeling alone or unsupported
(spiritual), and thinking that I'll be in pain every day (mental). I do
not abuse painkilling drugs such as opiates today, so I have learned
other strategies to deal with the pain. That leaves me with suffering,
which is the emotional component of pain. I understand and
accept my pain as a part of my life. I realize that in each life, pain
is inevitable; suffering, however, is optional. The choice is mine.
There are essentially two paths I can take. Neither eliminates pain,
but one path leads to healing and personal growth while the
other leads to ongoing suffering.

*I choose the path of personal growth and healing, knowing that
the opposite path leads to the use of painkilling drugs.*

HOPE

SPIRITUAL BALANCE

"Once you choose hope, anything is possible."
Unknown

Chronic pain causes physical suffering and distress. It is an ongoing and distressing sensation in a particular part of my body that aggravates and contributes to mental and emotional suffering or torment that inevitably accompanies my chronic pain. This combination creates spiritual imbalance. It is this spiritual imbalance that initially brings about feelings of hopelessness, low self-esteem, weakness, and lack of faith and connection to my Spirit, my higher power, and others. When I first realized that I would be living in chronic pain, quite possibly for the rest of my life, fear set in. I was left wondering what the rest of that life would be like. I projected a life based on how I felt the day I made that realization. In pain recovery I am challenged to accept my chronic pain, no longer fighting against it. I see my pain as something that makes me unique. From this, I develop strength, courage, hope, and greater faith that helps me to carry on each day.

I have hope for what tomorrow may look like, no matter how I'm feeling today. In pain recovery I have a reason to hope. Through twelve-step work and pain recovery, I search for peace, hope, strength, courage, and, of course, acceptance.

SICK ROLE

RELATIONSHIPS

"When someone in the family has chronic pain, family
roles and responsibilities often change, with the chronic
pain sufferer taking on a more dependent status or
sick role. My spouse or partner may take on too many
responsibilities if I'm in that role.... This role shift can lead to
feelings of resentment and frustration. The increased stress
on our relationship often leads to arguing or conflict, as
well as isolation, withdrawal, and even estrangement....
Because there is no end in sight for my chronic pain, I've
learned that the only way to truly deal with this situation
is by having honest and open communication.... No one
in the family needs to play the sick role and no one needs
to be the nurse or parent. The people in my family do not
need to be afraid that if they talk about their feelings they
are perceived as complaining or as a whiner."

Adapted from Pain Recovery: How to Find Balance
and Reduce Suffering from Chronic Pain

I may be in pain or physically sick, but that doesn't mean I have to
take on the "sick role" in my relationships. I make a contribution to
the household in whatever manner I can on any given day. I express
my concern and interest in how my family members are doing—I
don't just talk about me and my pain issues. In this way, I don't
become a burden—I remain a contributing member of the family.

*I give my family the dignity of seeing them as more than
just my caregivers—they are human beings in their own right,
with their own issues they sometimes need to share with me.
I am glad to be there for them.*

WILLINGNESS
PHYSICAL BALANCE

"No man ruleth safely but he that is willingly ruled."
Thomas à Kempis

It is much easier to practice willingness when I have some structure and routine in my day. It takes a long time to make a habit out of being healthy, and willingness is especially difficult if I'm having a particularly painful day. It's easier to practice willingness, putting one foot in front of the other, when I already have some kind of routine planned for that day. Pain recovery does not give me the luxury of being as spontaneous as I might like to be, or as I was in the past. In pain recovery I have to put a little more thought into a routine, building strong habits, so that when pain strikes—and it will—be it physical, emotional, or mental, I can practice willingness to get out of that pain, to have it lessened, by doing the next indicated right thing. The next right thing is usually the thing I had planned on doing before I was in pain, as if with the schedule, my healthy, happy, centered self was sending a message to the self in the future, saying, "This is what you need to do to help yourself so we can be back on track."

I send a message to my future self, who is experiencing pain, reminding that self of the things that need to be done for "us" to help us stay in pain recovery. Knowing that "bad days" will come, willingness is much easier to come by when there are some healthy habits I have formed in my program of pain recovery.

FAITH IN OTHERS

MENTAL BALANCE

....

"Let someone else drive. You may very well be
the better driver, and you may very well know the way,
but once in a while you need to experience
having faith in others."

The Soul Workout: Getting and Staying Spiritually Fit

Because I'm so familiar with my pain and know it better than
anyone else, I can fall into the trap of thinking I always know
what is best, for it and for me.

My ego can get in the way of my pain recovery when I insist that I
am right. I have to realize that the need and drive for pain relief can
sometimes skew my perceptions. In times like these, I need to take
a deep breath and listen to those around me who are my caregivers
and health providers. They have learned a thing or two about pain
recovery themselves. I need to maintain an open mind so that I can
have a new and perhaps better experience of pain recovery today.

I listen to others and take their loving advice as it is offered to me.

SPIRITUAL AWAKENING

EMOTIONAL BALANCE

....

"The emotions you often experience in your responses
to pain contribute to suffering; they contribute to the
hurt you feel from chronic pain."
A Day without Pain

In *Pain Recovery*, I learned about developing a new awareness.
This awareness is not something that is achieved and then set in
stone. It must change and grow as I do. I identify a source of pain
right now, at this moment. I get mad at it and tighten the muscles
in the area. I worry about how much worse it is getting, and throw
hatred right into the pain. I feel despair, because my mind tells
me this is the way it has always been, and even after all this
time the pain still hasn't gone anywhere. I hold these negative
feelings for a few moments.

Now I relax for a minute and take deep breaths. I set aside my angry
or despairing thoughts for a moment and just breathe. I loosen the
muscles that I tightened before and think about something positive.
I remember a favorite place, a song, a loved one—and relax.

*I write about the feelings that come up for me during my relaxation,
and compare them with the way I felt about this in the past.
I remember the techniques that I have developed and practice
them to help me shift my awareness.*

POWERLESSNESS

SPIRITUAL BALANCE

....

"Once members in a twelve-step program admit
their powerlessness over drugs or alcohol or food or sex
or gambling or whatever obsession in which they are
engaged, they are free to begin the recovery process.
This same principle can work for addressing your
chronic pain. You are powerless over your pain
and the circumstances that created it.
However, you are not helpless."
A Day without Pain

In the past, and even in recovery, my pain has caused
and does cause problems with my mobility. There were times
when I would focus so much upon the pain that it consumed me
mentally, spiritually, physically, and emotionally. These moments
left me with a complete feeling of powerlessness. But slowly in my
pain recovery I realized that powerless does not mean helpless.
In the First Step, I admit that I'm powerless over my addiction.
However, when I admit this, a power that I did not have before
flows into me. I continue to admit powerlessness over my addiction,
and by doing so, I'm able to achieve some measure of power
over my chronic pain.

*Through continuing to accept and be honest about my
powerlessness over addiction, I find power in my ability to live
a spiritually balanced life that makes it possible to live and enjoy
my life, even with chronic pain.*

AUGUST

11

GRATITUDE

RELATIONSHIPS

···

"Gratitude is the memory of the heart."
French proverb

Chronic pain teaches me lessons in gratitude. In the beginning, this may have been as simple as gratitude for days when my pain is not as bad as on other days, when I can function and be more mobile. Where I once might have been angry with the world or with God for what I have lost, I have learned to be grateful for what I have. If I find myself complaining because it is hard for me to get around, I need only to think of others whose circumstances are worse than my own, and look for opportunities to help them. I can channel my pain as a positive tool to help uplift the spirits of others who were once feeling as hopeless as I was. I may not have a choice in how my pain affects me physically, but I do have a choice in my emotional well-being. By embracing my pain as a part of my life instead of fighting against it, I am liberating myself. All the energy I once focused on why I hurt so badly is now positive energy that is turned toward helping those less fortunate than myself.

I will focus on doing something positive to help another person who is not as blessed as I am, and remember to give thanks for all that I have in my life.

ACCEPTANCE

PHYSICAL BALANCE

....

*"The acknowledgment of our weakness
is the first step in repairing our loss."*
Thomas à Kempis

Acceptance is not just a feeling; it is an action. To be in acceptance means creating habits in my life that are based on acknowledging my chronic pain and my commitment to recovery. Healthy habits include regularly meditating, exercising, attending recovery meetings, and continuing to work my pain recovery program.

Habits are not created overnight, nor are they things that are established and can then be left alone or unattended. In my physical pain, which needed, I felt, to be constantly nurtured, I created a habit of relying on friends and family in unhealthy ways. These habits have been replaced by healthy habits that are conducive to my pain recovery. But, to be in acceptance of my pain recovery, I must regularly monitor these new habits and renew my commitment to this new way of life of living with pain.

*I accept help from others today; I allow others to help me
ease my suffering from chronic pain. I am gracious in my acceptance,
letting those who offer assistance and support to feel my
appreciation and love.*

COMPASSION

MENTAL BALANCE

....

"It is lack of love for ourselves that inhibits our
compassion toward others. If we make friends
with ourselves, then there is no obstacle to opening
our hearts and minds to others."

Unknown

Living with chronic pain can cause me to feel isolated and
misunderstood. My pain may limit me physically, mentally,
emotionally, and spiritually on any given day. In the past, I used
this to draw pity from others, and I expected to receive compassion
from others that I know in retrospect I did not show to them.
Before I moved into a life of pain recovery, I expected others—
doctors, pharmacists, therapists—to be accountable for my pain.
Through working the steps and staying in recovery, today
I take responsibility for myself.

Having compassion for others, rather than expecting it from
them, takes the focus off my own pain, reducing its intensity, and
ironically, I usually find the compassion from others I was seeking
all along when I try to be a little more compassionate toward them.

*I accept help gratefully from those who are compassionate enough
to help me. Some people have been kind enough to help me despite
their own problems. I do what I can for myself, and show my
appreciation to those who help me.*

SELF-CARE

EMOTIONAL BALANCE

....

*"Taking some time each day to write about your
journey can help you identify thought patterns, express
feelings, maintain gratitude, and monitor progress."*
Pain Recovery: How to Find Balance and
Reduce Suffering from Chronic Pain

The manifestations of my chronic pain include feelings of
depression, anger, worry, discouragement, and irritability. If I
am feeling any of these feelings in recovery, I need to pay special
attention. In recovery, I do not have the luxury of letting these
feelings go unchecked. I must talk to someone in my pain recovery
support group. I must journal about these feelings. I must talk to my
sponsor. More importantly, I must not let these feelings become an
excuse to stay down, stay home, and fall back into old patterns.

Granted, I have bad days and good days during which different
feelings come up. But how long do those feelings last? Has this
been going on for days, or weeks? Am I taking action in my recovery
regardless of how I am feeling? As long as I am focusing on my
recovery, feelings come and go. But I am not my feelings—they are
just something that I experience and from which I can move on.

*I pay attention to my feelings because they are a tool I can use to
know where I am in my chronic pain and my recovery. I do not let my
feelings decide what I am doing or not doing for my recovery.*

ACCEPTANCE

SPIRITUAL BALANCE

....

*"For after all, the best thing one can do
when it's raining is to let it rain."*
Henry Wadsworth Longfellow

I sometimes underestimate the power of acceptance. This principle tends to be the most gratifying, as well as giving me the peace of mind for which I have been striving for a very long time. Living with my pain on a daily basis, I tend to struggle with the concept of acceptance. How can I live in acceptance if this is never going to change? How am I going to be able to live life when I hurt so bad? What kind of life will I have if this pain never goes away? How can I truly be kind to others with the way I feel? These and numerous other questions go through my head on a daily basis. These are self-defeating thoughts, and as long as I tantalize myself with these questions, I never find any kind of peace of mind in my life. The meaning of true acceptance is to be practiced on a daily basis. I know that whatever pain I am going through, I am okay—no matter what. Acceptance is universal and can be used in every situation that arises. If I truly grasp the concept of acceptance, then maybe, just maybe, I'll find true peace in my life no matter how bad my pain is.

I strive to live in acceptance. I look at the positive things that the day brings and don't dwell on the negative.

JOY AND FREEDOM

RELATIONSHIPS

"Joy shared is joy doubled."
Swedish proverb

I've been through a lot during this journey with chronic pain. Now that I'm in pain recovery I look forward to a life of joy and freedom from the constant worry of how much pain certain activities might cause. I've also learned a lot on this journey, and when I look back on where I've come from I take the lessons learned and give them away freely to another. These lessons are often universal, applying broadly to the human condition. So while I have learned them because of my chronic pain recovery, perhaps I can help others with the same care and compassion that has been shown to me, whether they too suffer from chronic pain or not. My higher power reminds me that we are all interconnected, that just as I need to find the humility to accept help from another, I must find the courage to give back to others when the opportunity arises.

I remain observant for the opportunity to help another who may be struggling.

AMENDS

PHYSICAL BALANCE

···

"If you bring forth what is within you, what you bring
forth will save you. If you do not bring forth what is within
you, what you do not bring forth will destroy you."
Jesus Christ, the Gospel of Thomas

Amends are a powerful tool in my pain recovery. I must take action
to make amends to those I have harmed. Emotional pain weighs
heavily on my conscience and contributes to my chronic pain. I do
not allow emotional pain to weigh on my conscience and cause me
pain or threaten my recovery. To avoid unnecessary stress (and pain)
I make amends to those I have harmed. I do so in a thoughtful and
considerate manner, with the guidance of my sponsor. I do not
cause further harm. I understand that those I have harmed may not
want to participate in my quest to make amends.

*I use the tools of my recovery and the advice of my sponsor to maintain
a clean slate and to make amends for my past wrongs. When I need to,
I make amends with the guidance of my sponsor, and remember that
the best amends are sometimes simply the effort to "amend" my life.*

STRENGTH

MENTAL BALANCE

....

"Our strength grows out of our weakness."
Ralph Waldo Emerson

Pain recovery is a lifelong journey. I have chronic pain today, but as my recovery progresses I learn new tools for managing pain. Each day brings new understanding of what works and what doesn't. When I focus on the solutions that my recovery has given me, I get the strength to live with my pain, allowing it to be part of me rather than something I fight against.

Strength does not just mean that I am able to lift more, do more, or handle more. Sometimes strength is admitting I can handle less. Strength is the ability to do what it is within my means to do, whether that's less or more than I'd like to do. Strength is accepting my limitations, but not being a victim of my limitations. Strength is acceptance. Strength is courage to go on another day, attend another meeting, help another person. Strength is living life without the abuse of medication, continuing to build an arsenal of tools that help me lessen the intensity of my pain and increase my tolerance for it. Strength is crying and laughter. Strength is thinking, holding the thought in my mind that I am capable and strong, that I am in recovery and living life with chronic pain today, not dying from chronic pain. Strength is a mental investment in my well-being, healing, and love.

I find my strength and mental focus when I think on the solutions pain recovery has granted me thus far. Strength in mind comes from my continuous search, looking forward to the new lessons and tools I learn today that will help me tomorrow.

STRENGTH

EMOTIONAL BALANCE

"Dwell not upon thy weariness; thy strength shall be
according to the measure of thy desire."
Arab proverb

I once thought of strength only in terms of physical endurance. However, my mental, emotional, and moral strength are also important contributors to my pain recovery. Mental strength (toughness) is my ability to accept pain as a necessary part of life and to follow the necessary steps to reach my goals. Emotional strength is my ability to keep my emotions in check. I cannot react to pain in a negative manner. Moral strength or strength of character is my ability to do what is right. To do what is right allows me to maintain a clear conscience. A clear conscience allows me to greet each day with renewed optimism. Strength comes in many forms and expressions. My ability to exhibit strength in all areas of my life allows me to view my pain in a proper perspective and to continue my recovery. Strength is an asset, and my willingness and ability to build assets in recovery are essential to my continued success.

*I discover where I am strong and where I can become stronger.
I exhibit strength in all areas of my life.*

MY LEARNING
SPIRITUAL BALANCE

....

"Much learning does not teach understanding."
Heraclitus

Even though I might feel I have learned everything I can to
deal with my pain, I'll never reach my full potential if I do not
continue the journey forward with the goal of achieving greater
understanding. I strive to learn something new every day. If I don't,
then I won't keep progressing. Eventually, I'll lose all the gifts I've
gained. I know I've acquired numerous tools to deal with my pain.
I have a great deal of peace in my life. However, I have something
inside me always yearning to learn more, do more, and be more.
The only way I know how to accomplish this is to stay open-minded
and humble on a daily basis no matter who crosses my path.
That is the way to spiritual balance for me.

*Even though I may have some physical and emotional relief
from my pain today that does not mean I have learned everything
there is to learn about my recovery. I continue to strive for new
solutions, new answers, and a new way of life, so someday I can
reach my full potential.*

DISCOVERY

RELATIONSHIPS

"All truths are easy to understand once they are
discovered; the point is to discover them."
Galileo Galilei

I've discovered many truths in my recovery, including the
correlation among my relationships, my ability to live with my
pain, and my quality of life. I've discovered through the process
of working the Twelve Steps, talking to my sponsor, working with
others, and being an active participant in my own life and the
lives of those around me that the relationships I have are a direct
reflection of my spiritual state and my connection to a higher
power. On days when I struggle with my relationships, pain may be
amplified. When I'm in pain and become irritable or unreasonable
with the relationships in my life, I can use my pain to justify my
behavior. What I cannot justify is knowing that there's a better
way to live and yet not living that way.

*I remember to treat others as if it's a good day every day, whether
I'm in pain or not. I value the relationships in my life, treating others
with patience, kindness, and tolerance.*

ATTITUDE

PHYSICAL BALANCE

....

"Whenever you're in conflict with someone,
there is one factor that can make the difference
between damaging your relationship and deepening it.
That factor is attitude."

William James

Am I in the habit of monitoring my attitude? Do I take time
to look at my attitude toward life and recovery? Whatever my
attitude is on any given day, over a period of time it can improve.
Because of my history, I do not have the luxury of letting my
attitude and outlook on life go unchecked. Knowing this helps me
commit to the habit of taking my own inventory and making sure
that my attitude is not one that leads me to states of mind that I
know are not good for me. I maintain an "attitude of gratitude"
for the things that I'm able to accomplish today, and reject the
negativity that can come when I dwell on the things I cannot do.
When I have a conflict, I may not be able to change the other
person's mind, but I can change my attitude.

My daily life is better when I get into the habit of monitoring
my attitude, and making positive adjustments as needed.

NOTICING MY THOUGHTS

MENTAL BALANCE

....

"The unexamined life is not worth living."
Socrates

Pain recovery includes working on consciously restructuring my thought process to allow for acknowledgment and recognition of my thoughts without overreacting to them. Slowing down the thought process is the beginning of this new habit and helps me move toward balance. Instead of identifying my thoughts as indisputable facts, I allow myself to observe them with interest and curiosity. With practice, I have been able to witness my thoughts as they arise in my awareness.

I slow down and observe my thoughts. I take a few moments to observe my thoughts as they come up for me in the moment. I take a little time each day to practice this slowing-down strategy. I write about this daily in a journal or notebook. I reflect on what I have written, and look at how I've grown.

I mind the way I think in every part of my life. I become aware of the way I may distort messages I receive from others depending on my pain level on any given day. I slow down and remind myself to think positively.

RECOVERY

EMOTIONAL BALANCE

....

"I am free from active addiction and experience the relief from having to use drugs to live with chronic pain. By working the Twelve Steps, I have found that anything is possible. The only limits to my recovery from addiction and chronic pain exist in my head."

Pain Recovery: How to Find Balance and
Reduce Suffering from Chronic Pain

When I'm feeling good, it seems like anything is possible—then I hit a wall. It could be due to an injury from some activity; it could be because my family isn't doing what I want them to at the moment, or because someone has spoken to me "the wrong way." No matter what has happened to put me into a bad mood, I remember to be grateful that today I'm free from active addiction. Numbing out with drugs may once have seemed like a solution; however, life has a tendency to go on around me, and any problems I used to think I'd escaped only compounded, magnified, progressed, and then became ten times worse later on, when I would come out of my fog.

Regardless of what I'm feeling, recovery continues as long as I keep my head "in the game." How do I do this? I take the focus off negative thoughts and feelings by doing the "next right thing." I may feel sad, bad, or any other negative feeling, but if I keep moving through my program of recovery, my thoughts and feelings will not have the power over me that they once had.

I have a program of recovery and that gives me the freedom to live life—to take the good along with the bad, and have a life worth living.

KINDNESS

SPIRITUAL BALANCE

"Whether we ever see a response or whether the
response is immediate or delayed, there is a benefit
to kindness in our lives and in the lives of others."
Of Character: Building Assets in Recovery

Outward acts of kindness have a direct effect on my spiritual
inner life and connectedness to my higher power. I believe my
higher power is loving and kind, and I act the way I believe my
higher power would have me act toward others. Acting in this way
manifests a healing power within me, and my physical body draws
on this inner strength. The more I act in kindness—the more
I act in the will of a higher, loving power—the more reserves I store
inside myself on a spiritual-healing level. These reserves will
be called upon when my chronic pain flares up. It is not a
question of *if*, but *when* I need that strength.

*In pain recovery, I don't wait until I need healing, loving energy
from my inner self to fill myself with healing, loving energy. The energy
I call upon for my own well-being increases with every act of kindness
I extend to another human being.*

CATASTROPHIZING

PHYSICAL BALANCE

....

"There is no quick fix. Changes are most effective when
they are incremental changes. I consider all four points
of balance: physical, emotional, mental, and spiritual.
Imbalance often results from being unduly harsh and
mentally catastrophizing, so I resist the urge to become
discouraged, punish, blame, feel shame, or overreact."

*Pain Recovery: How to Find Balance and
Reduce Suffering from Chronic Pain*

All four points represent the whole of my life and recovery. I view
them as connected, and I deal with them collectively. I have
regard for the big picture, so that when something happens in
one area I don't lose focus on the other areas of my life. Often
when I experience a problem—such as a relationship problem or
a problems at work—I don't catastrophize the situation as I used
to do. There was a time when a disagreement with my romantic
partner would seem like the end of the relationship, and a missed
deadline or quota at work had me thinking ahead to losing my job,
becoming homeless, and sleeping under a bridge!

I don't catastrophize today—instead, I focus on my physical,
emotional, mental, and spiritual balance. I focus on the healthy
and recovery-oriented habits I know work for me, allowing time to
work in my favor in the other "problem" areas of my life.

*When something does not go my way, I do not make a big deal out of it
or focus too much attention on it—instead, I focus on the four points of
balance and the healthy habits and techniques I've learned in recovery.*

APPLYING THE
SERENITY PRAYER

MENTAL BALANCE

"It's one thing to pray, another to actually
apply the Serenity Prayer."
Of Character: Building Assets in Recovery

The Serenity Prayer is more than just something I can say in the mornings, during the day, or at meetings. In the prayer there is a way for me to live. I can identify something related to my pain condition that I cannot change and need to accept. Perhaps I've been working hard on a particular area of my body but it just won't seem to cooperate. No matter how much physical therapy or exercise I do, I just can't seem to make a breakthrough in this area, and my pain level remains about the same. It's important when this happens to identify something about the condition that I *can* change. Perhaps it's just my response to it. I want it to change so much that I'm actually causing part of the problem. So I say the Serenity Prayer, and change what I can. With the help of my sponsor, counselor, therapist, doctors, support group members and my higher power, I begin to identify differences in those things that I can change.

I relate the Serenity Prayer to what is troubling in my life and walk through the process of how it relates to me today.

NONJUDGMENTAL

EMOTIONAL BALANCE

....

*"Sometimes you may think
that you shouldn't feel the way you do."*
Pain Recovery: How to Find Balance and
Reduce Suffering from Chronic Pain

I don't judge my emotions today. Instead I remember that
feelings aren't facts, and they don't need "fixing." That's a new
way of thinking for me.

My old way of thinking about my feelings used to go something like
this: "Oh-oh! Anxiety! That's bad, right? Oh, well, I can't have anxiety,
so I need to 'fix' that right now!" Of course, the quickest and easiest
way for me to "fix" my feelings was to use. A drug might "fix"
my immediate emotional or physical pain—in the short run.
However, the overall and ultimate damage it would do to my life
would have much worse results.

Today, I remember that I'm human, and so sometimes I'm going to
have feelings that I do not like. I remind myself that I have no problem
when happiness arises, seemingly without reason, so I shouldn't have
a problem with anxiety, fear, sadness, or any other "negative" emotion
that arises. Although these emotions are unpleasant, I can face them
today with my program and fellowship of pain recovery.

*Today I avoid judging my feelings as good or bad. I use the tools of recovery
to get "out of myself" and do the next right thing, changing the focus from
worry over feelings I once judged as bad to actions I can take that relieve
my negative feelings. I can find a solution in my recovery program.*

ACCEPTANCE
SPIRITUAL BALANCE

....

"Acceptance of what has happened is the first step to
overcoming the consequences of any misfortune."
William James

Sometimes life brings me great joy and other times it brings me
great sorrow. Through acceptance I'm able to take the good with
the bad. If I had no pain I would not appreciate pleasure. Pain
allows me to better understand and accept my inner self. Through
acceptance I'm able to strive for balance physically, mentally,
emotionally, and spiritually. I accept the fact that when I'm
suffering from pain it's because I'm not in balance.

I accept the fact that the pain I feel may be a direct result of my
past action or inaction. Perhaps pain exists to move me to action.
If I choose inaction instead of action, I cannot expect positive
results. Recovery does not just require action—recovery *is* action.

*I understand that through acceptance I am better able to master my
pain and to experience a greater sense of balance. Acceptance and
balance are therefore two ways to reduce pain and eliminate suffering.
Acceptance prompts action. Action produces results. Results are
what pain recovery is all about.*

SOLUTION TO SUFFERING

RELATIONSHIPS

....

"Have compassion for all beings, rich and poor alike;
each has their suffering. Some suffer too much,
others too little."

Siddhartha Gautama, the Buddha

When I'm suffering with chronic pain it's easy to feel I'm alone and
have no one to reach out to. But in recovery I realize I'm not alone.
Many suffer from chronic pain and are in pain recovery. These
others are a source of comfort and strength.

By reaching out to others with chronic pain who are in recovery,
I find a way to focus more on them and less on myself, and that
includes focusing less on my own perceived suffering. In my
relationships with others, I discover peace and serenity.

Living with chronic pain is an ongoing learning experience. When
my mind is wandering back to the edges of the storm, I focus my
thoughts back to the center: prayer, meetings, steps, sponsors,
therapists, writing, reading, meditating, exercising, and not abusing
medication, no matter what.

*Through the process of reaching out, I move to the eye of the storm
that is within me. I'm relieved of the mental burden of feeling alone,
isolated, depressed, and despairing. Through reaching out, my mind
can focus instead on the strength of others who have walked this path
before me, with me, and who will follow after.*

FAITH

PHYSICAL BALANCE

....

"The feeling remains that God is on the journey, too."
St. Teresa of Avila

Some in recovery say a person can't actually be in fear and in faith at the same time. Others have a different saying that expresses a similar idea: "If you're gonna worry about it—don't bother to pray about it. If you're gonna *pray* about it—then don't worry about it." Still others express it this way: "Pray for help, than act as if it's on its way."

After a lifetime spent trying to manage my own life, convinced that I knew best and that if only I could figure out a better way to "do it," I could continue in my addiction without any negative consequences, I had to reach out in faith to a higher power. And then I had to get out of His way, trust that He cared for me and only wanted good things for me, and trust that if I asked Him for help, it would come. No worries. My higher power is with me every step of the way on my journey of recovery. All I have to do is ask for help and it will come.

Considering the scientific evidence that worry worsens chronic pain and contributes to other physical conditions, I maintain my physical balance by this spiritual means: I stop worrying and take my problems to my higher power to solve. I am powerless, but He has all the power in the world. All I need to do is accept His will for me.

I am on a journey with my higher power today. My faith sends a message to my body, mind, and spirit that I'm in recovery and planning to stay that way with the help of my higher power.

{ S E P T E M B E R }

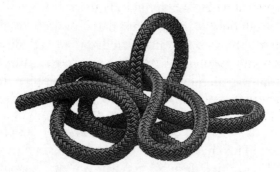

EXPECTATIONS

MENTAL BALANCE

....

"Expectations kill."
The Soul Workout: Getting and Staying Spiritually Fit

It's not what life throws at me that challenges me so much as it is the discrepancy between what life throws at me and what I thought I wanted from life. As a human being I have natural desires and needs that I'd like to have fulfilled. That's perfectly normal.

My problems begin when I start expecting certain outcomes from my actions instead of just doing the next right thing and then accepting my higher power's will for me. When I start fantasizing about getting what I want out of life—money, power, prestige, possessions, or what have you—then I stop living in the now. I miss out on the beauty today has to offer. And I set myself up for disappointment when my needs are not met, as they rarely can be. After all, how can anyone else meet the extravagant needs that I can fabricate in my mind? They can't. Nor should I expect them to. No one else is here to meet my expectations, and that's quite freeing— it means I'm not here to meet anyone else's expectations, either.

I'm just here to "do the footwork," and leave the results up to my higher power.

LOVE

EMOTIONAL BALANCE

"What does love look like? It has the hands to help others.
It has the feet to hasten to the poor and needy. It has the
eyes to see misery and want. It has the ears to hear the
sighs and sorrows of men. That is what love looks like."
Saint Augustine

There is a world of difference between "being in love" as depicted
in movies, poetry, songs, and novels and truly loving myself and
others. The "in-love feeling" is infatuation, mostly based on
how that other person makes me feel.

The love I seek in recovery is the feeling that comes *after* the
infatuation I feel for another person—it's not the butterflies in
the stomach, the sweaty palms, or the lack of sleep. Love is the
extension of myself for the betterment of another, putting myself in
his or her shoes and treating that person as I'd want to be treated.
Love is doing things that are caring and nurturing, and that take
another's needs into consideration, putting my body, mind, and
spirit at their service. Love is an action word—and when I take that
action, the feelings of love naturally follow. I do not wait to first
have the feeling of love in order to act, because my understanding
of love is distorted by years of chronic pain and active addiction.
Instead of waiting for the feeling, I take loving action.
That is love to me today.

*Love drives away pain—the love I show to others, and the love I accept
from them, too; the love of being alive and part of the circle of life.
Love washes over me and dissolves some of the pain I feel right now.*

FLOW, FLUX

SPIRITUAL BALANCE

"He who grasps things loses them."
Lao Tzu

I sometimes achieve balance only for a fleeting moment. Some days, it seems I do nothing but pass from one extreme to another. As I move all too quickly past the point of balance, I swing to another extreme. Prayer and meditation, focusing on my breathing, and calming my mind can restore me to a place of balance in a day when my pain threatens to become extreme. I go with the flow of my life today—not clutching desperately at moments of happiness, but letting go and letting my higher power provide for my needs.

Accepting that some days I will experience movements from one extreme to another is vital to achieving spiritual balance. I allow myself to experience the process of recovery. I don't try to grasp and hold the pleasant feelings that accompany balance; I accept that I am a work in progress, always in flux. I accept that I need to work on a certain area—such as regular prayer and meditation—and start today. By accepting the need for this process as part of my program of recovery, I'm ready and able to accept the fact of my pain and find the balance necessary to recover.

I accept that balance requires work, and that work doesn't mean I have to be hard on myself—it just means accepting that spiritual balance is a flow, requiring adjustment, like a dance. I'm doing the dance of recovery—instead of the dance of death—with my disease today.

REACHING OUT

RELATIONSHIPS

....

"Solitude vivifies; isolation kills."
Joseph Roux

Like many people, I live with many types of pain in my life: emotional, chronic, or acute, with chronic pain often being the most prevailing. Regardless of the type of pain, when I'm in any kind of pain my first instinct is to push everyone away. I don't want to talk or listen. In isolation, I hurt only myself—and sometimes it seems that's just what I want to do. I look at my behavior and wonder what am I getting out of acting this way?

Pain, misery, and addiction served me with secondary benefits such as the sympathy of others and the opportunity to shirk responsibility. Eventually, though, those secondary benefits disappeared, as that behavior left me (and can leave me, even in recovery) isolated and lonely. I've learned tools in pain recovery that have helped me deal with all types of pain; I no longer need to manipulate or isolate to achieve secondary gains that don't work for me in the long run.

With recovery tools in hand, I have the ability to reach out, even when I don't want to. I know that reaching out to others to obtain help with the solution and my recovery is far more important than reaching out to get sympathy or enabling. I reach out and trust others who have gone through similar pain.

SEPTEMBER

5

FLEXIBILITY

PHYSICAL BALANCE

....

*"We are all bound to the throne of the Supreme Being
by a flexible chain which restrains without enslaving us.
The most wonderful aspect of the universal
scheme of things is the action of free beings
under divine guidance."*
Joseph de Maistre

Tomorrow builds upon whatever I do today. I will feel the results of whatever I do today tomorrow, no matter which of the points of balance I am focusing on. Physically, I work every day at becoming more flexible and increasing my mobility, ability, and function. Am I stretching today? Have I gone to yoga? Am I doing the exercises that were recommended by my physical therapist or doctor?

I continually monitor my ability to be flexible and monitor my pain. If I'm performing a certain stretch and my pain level is a six, but a month or even a year ago it was a seven, then I'm recovering—I'm getting better. I need not be discouraged, but must always work on increasing my physical flexibility as I progress through my program of recovery, mindful that flexibility has its applications in every area of my life, the mental, emotional, and spiritual as well as the physical.

*I make sure I'm working on my flexibility. I stretch, go to yoga,
or work with my doctor or therapist to make sure I'm making progress
in this area, knowing that I'm either moving forward or moving
backward. I choose to move forward.*

EXTREMES OF THINKING

MENTAL BALANCE

....

"In everything the middle course is best;
all things in excess bring trouble."
Plautus

I pay attention to and consider my different styles of thinking—
sometimes I minimize actions and events, and at other times
I spend too much time and energy analyzing, intellectualizing,
or rationalizing my feelings and behavior. If I "under" think, I may
react to situations immediately, emotionally and impulsively, rather
than by thinking logically and acting based on consideration of the
needs of the situation and selecting from available options I have
today in recovery. Today I avoid extremes.

I value my ideas as much as I value my feelings. I approach
situations mindfully and try to find logical solutions to issues that
arise, but I don't ignore my feelings, either. Sometimes it's a "gut
feeling" that keeps me away from "slippery" places, persons, or
things. I could rationalize or think my way into those places, but by
maintaining an open channel among the four points of balance,
I find the right course of action for me today.

I pay attention to any extreme thinking I may have, and talk about
this with my sponsor or counselor. What areas of my life may I be
under- or over-thinking? Am I ignoring my feelings or intuitions by
retreating into intellectualization? I strive for balance between
too much and not enough.

JOY

EMOTIONAL BALANCE

"When the mind is pure,
joy follows like a shadow that never leaves."
Siddhartha Gautama, the Buddha

My emotional responses to situations are often just learned behaviors, which in the process of pain recovery I've been systematically relearning—remolding my "plastic brain." In the course of that hard-wiring and rewiring, I strive to hard-wire getting in touch with my joy in being alive. I hope that joy is the first response in waking up and finding myself alive and in recovery each day. I want to react to every situation in life with that response. This is an ideal that I may never actually achieve, but I can think on it, meditate on it, and imagine what it would be like. I can act *as if* until it actually happens. When I get in touch with the joy I have for my life—even for my pain, because it is a part of me— I reprogram my mind and consequently change my emotional responses to situations.

I respond with joy first. I allow joy to come into my mind, and then allow the joy in my mind to influence my emotions, feelings, and responses. I understand this takes time and practice, and I am joyful about that as well.

HOPE

SPIRITUAL BALANCE

....

"Recovery plants the seed of hope in all who
choose to stay and grow. It is the sapling that
struggles to touch the sun each day."
Tails of Recovery: Addicts and the Pets That Love Them

The sapling stretches toward, but will never actually touch, the
sun. I will never be completely free of chronic pain. As the leaves
of a sapling absorb the sunlight, I absorb the healing energy of
pain recovery. The sunlight turns into the nourishment and energy
so the seed may one day turn into a tree. The Twelve Steps of
recovery provide me the nourishment to one day heal and grow
into a person who has made a life worth living, even with chronic
pain. My struggles turn into hope. Where once my pain seemed so
overwhelming, so daunting, so impossible, it is that hope that helps
me grow into the person who can live life without abusing pain
medication. I can provide hope for others. They see me standing
tall, having gone through so many growing pains, so many days
of seeing a little spot in the sky millions of miles away, but I keep
reaching, keep stretching, keep hoping. Hope turns to faith and
trust. Hope stems from desire.

My desire to grow in recovery is my root system; hope forms my
branches, stretching and spreading into the sky, where they will provide
shade and shelter for my fellow creatures one day.

APPRECIATION

RELATIONSHIPS

....

"O Divine Master, grant that I may not so much seek to
be consoled as to console;
to be understood as to understand;
to be loved as to love."

St. Francis of Assisi

My pain caused me to push people away if I felt they didn't understand
me sufficiently, or couldn't appreciate what I was experiencing. It
was impossible for me to believe that people—even those close to
me, who I knew loved me—really understood what I was going
through. Looking back, I wonder why I was so intent on having others
understand me and my pain. As I considered this, I realized that I was
seeing others as mirrors that I believed should only reflect me—my
thoughts, my feelings, and my pain. I was treating others as "less than,"
and myself as the only one who mattered. What a waste.

Today I know that it is more important in my recovery for me to
try to understand others than to attempt to have them understand
me. I show appreciation for others and their struggles, which today
I realize are just as significant to them as mine are to me. I seek
to "console" rather than to be consoled. And in doing so, I find
consolation and strengthened relationships are my reward.

*Today I find consolation and meaning in helping others, whereas
I once thought only of how others could help me. I speak softly, if at
all, of any pain, and then only to acquire any necessary help—not
to vent my frustration or anger. I gain serenity in proportion to the
degree to which I help others today.*

GRATITUDE
PHYSICAL BALANCE

"Gratitude of character starts with a profound, often reverent appreciation of what we have been given. It extends to the action we take to honor that feeling."
Of Character: Building Assets in Recovery

In pain recovery I have to make a habit of demonstrating my gratitude. If I don't use it, I'll lose it—this is how my body works. I'm grateful that I have function and ability, in whatever capacity that is, and I show my gratitude by using my body in whatever way it can and will be used. If I can walk, I show my gratitude for that ability by walking. If I can do yoga, work out with weights, run, play sports of any kind, I do so.

This is a far cry from where I was when I was stuck in bed, hopelessly addicted to pain medication, unable to even hold conversations let alone get out of the house and do anything physical. I also make a habit of showing my gratitude by continuing to attend meetings, no matter how I'm feeling, whether good or not so good, showing my gratitude to those who helped me by showing up. Just showing up with a willing heart can be a way of expressing my gratitude. I make a habit of doing chores in the household, being part of that little community. I do not need to always tell people how I'm feeling, but show them my gratitude by my regular habits.

I show gratitude for my body, its function, and for those in my life and recovery network by making it a habit to do things I might not have been able to normally do for fear of the pain it once caused.

SENSE OF PROPORTION

MENTAL BALANCE

....

"With mental balance, I challenge the assumptions
I have about my pain. My pain is neither the worst
that ever happened nor is it insignificant. It is not a
punishment; it is simply an occurrence in the course
of life that has various challenging ripple effects."

Pain Recovery: How to Find Balance and
Reduce Suffering from Chronic Pain

I know I have a tendency to overdramatize, and not just my pain.
Sometimes when I'm talking to someone, I have to stop and laugh at
myself, because I realize that the scenario I'm describing, which may
have happened to me or to someone else, is taking on epic proportions
as I speak. Everything that has ever happened to me, it seems, is either
the best or the worst, the most comical or the most tragic. Sure, it
makes for an entertaining story—but is it really so epic?

A sense of proportion is important in all things, but especially in
dealing with my chronic pain and my recovery. I'm neither the
best nor the worst, neither a "ten" nor a "two"—I'm happy to be
a "five" today, in the middle of the herd, where I am safe in my
recovery fellowship. It's fun to be the center of attention sometimes,
but I keep a sense of proportion, and stop dramatizing my life—
especially when it comes to my chronic pain.

*A balanced mental attitude helps me keep my "tragedies"
and "triumphs" in proportion. My pain is not the slightest, nor
is it the most intolerable. It just is. I have tools today to deal with
my pain that make it tolerable.*

FORGIVENESS

EMOTIONAL BALANCE

"Humanity is never so beautiful as when praying
for forgiveness, or else forgiving another."
Jean Paul Richter

It's okay for me to be sad about the pain that I'm in, but I need to
be careful not to let that sadness slip into self-pity or despair. When
I'm sad or upset about the things that have happened to my body,
I remember that it's not my body's fault. I am conscious of the
fact that chronic pain is something that millions of other people
have for a variety of reasons. I forgive my body, and through that
forgiveness I have empathy for my body rather than pity or despair.
I send love to those areas of my body that hurt, rather than negative
emotions such as anger, sorrow, regret, pity, or sadness. I view my
pain with love, compassion, and forgiveness.

Regardless of the way my chronic pain came to be a part
of my life, I remember that life happens, pain happens, and I have
the ability to recover. It doesn't matter what I did or how I got
to where I am. I forgive myself and remember it's about where
I'm going that matters.

*I forgive my body for the pain I have been in. I call on the
positive feelings I've learned in recovery and direct them to those
parts of my body that hurt today.*

BELIEF

SPIRITUAL BALANCE

"Pray, and row the boat."
American proverb

I say I "believe" in a higher power, and my program of recovery teaches me that this higher power can restore me to sanity. But I must back up my beliefs with actions. I take action to preserve my spiritual balance, even during those "dark nights of the soul" when actual "belief," as in a comforting and unshakable faith, seems far away. This is one of many ways I have today to build my spiritual strength and achieve spiritual balance. I pray to my higher power, but I row my boat toward the shore of recovery.

I take loving actions and conduct all my affairs in the belief that spiritual balance is possible when I live my program in the emotional, mental, and physical dimensions of my existence and in all my relationships with others.

STRENGTH

RELATIONSHIPS

....

"Our strength grows out of our weaknesses."
Ralph Waldo Emerson

Pain has not always led me down the easiest of paths.
Sometimes simple chores or outings require extra effort, time,
or strength. As a person living with chronic pain, I remember that
my body has its limitations as well as its strengths. I neither diminish
my strengths nor magnify my weaknesses. I give each the proper
regard and respect.

An old Irish proverb says, "God makes the back for the burden."
I take this to mean that as my higher power has created me, so He
knows how much I can handle. Although it may seem to me at
times that my burden of pain is more than I can stand, I remember
that in actuality it isn't. I can call on my higher power for strength,
not only to endure, but to persevere, and to make a positive
contribution to the lives of those around me.

I have an important role to play amongst my friends and loved ones.
My pain does not make me helpless, nor does it diminish my value
to those who love me and those whom I love.

MAINTENANCE

PHYSICAL BALANCE

"(The body is) a marvelous machine...a chemical laboratory, a power-house. Every movement, voluntary or involuntary, is full of secrets and marvels!"
Theodor Herzl

Physical balance requires me to be mindful and respectful of my body, which includes paying attention to the messages it sends to my brain. I evaluate the state of my body thoroughly and continually, without becoming preoccupied. "How am I feeling? If there is pain, where is it coming from and how bad is it? What action that has worked in the past might I take to modify it—stretch, change position, get up and move, breathe, listen to soothing music, talk to someone (reach out), or share with someone who is hurting more (give back)?"

With physical balance, I have an organized series of maintenance and crisis interventions. For example, a good maintenance regimen that keeps my pain tolerable consists of regular exercise, meditation, getting massages, stretching, and chiropractic, in addition to taking balancing actions that I learned in *Pain Recovery*.

I have a good maintenance program. If I'm regularly maintaining my life and recovery, then I may not be entirely rid of my pain today, but I know that I can live without being addicted to medications that inhibit my life and make it difficult to live a happy, productive existence.

16

EXTREME NEGATIVE THINKING

MENTAL BALANCE

"The other side of the spectrum from extreme positive thinking is extreme negative thinking. Negative thinking is walking around thinking everything is lousy and always will be, regardless of what happens. Chronic negative thinking actually makes bad situations worse. When I'm thinking negatively I tend to ruminate, going over and over situations in my mind, playing the same scene over and over, unproductively. I'm not thinking about how I could have handled something better. I'm not being in a solution. Instead, I'm focused on everything that's wrong. I magnify the negative and exaggerate the significance of something that occurred, turning what was really only a small problem into a major disaster in my mind. My thoughts have the capacity to make my life miserable. Negative thinking can be especially insidious, feeding on itself, with the potential to become a self-fulfilling prophecy."

Pain Recovery: How to Find Balance and
Reduce Suffering from Chronic Pain

Thinking may or may not take me to extremes, but having chronic pain or addiction or both typically includes experiencing various degrees of distorted, out-of-balance thinking. Imbalance in thinking can cause imbalances in emotional, physical, and spiritual functioning. Today I keep my thinking balanced between positive and negative.

Am I magnifying the negative and diminishing the positive today?
Or am I making an effort to see things as they really are, in balance,
remembering always that it really is not "all about me"?

FLEXIBILITY

EMOTIONAL BALANCE

"Blessed are the flexible,
for they can tie themselves into knots."
Unknown

An aspect of emotional maturity in recovery is the ability to be flexible. While I've had to make strides physically by exercising, stretching, and focusing on the flexibility of my body, I've also had to work on mental flexibility by being open-minded to another process for handling my pain. Spiritual flexibility has come (and continues to come) through working steps, counseling, meetings, prayer, and meditation.

Emotional flexibility is about accepting my feelings as they emerge, being careful to remember that I am not my feelings, any more than I am my pain. Just because I have a feeling about something in particular does not mean that I need to react. I remember that sometimes my emotions are fueled or aggravated by my pain, just as my thinking is capable of making my emotions seem intolerable. In pain recovery, I have the flexibility to "go with the flow" and allow the feelings that I have to come and go. Without flexibility I have no chance of moving from a negative or unhappy feeling to a feeling of acceptance, hope, and happiness. In pain recovery I must always stay flexible in my body, mind, and spirit. Only through flexibility am I able to get outside a comfort zone that at one point before recovery was a distorted comfort with the pain and lifestyle I was living while abusing medication and living in active addiction.

I observe my feelings and invite flexibility into my life, allowing myself to move and shift from one feeling to another without necessarily reacting to any of the feelings that I have.

COMMITMENT

SPIRITUAL BALANCE

"Being committed requires the consistency
and fortitude to do what is required even when
we are tired or don't feel we can."
Of Character: Building Assets in Recovery

When the pain was too much to handle, I abandoned myself by
abusing medication and living in active addiction. My recovery
is a commitment to myself. It is a commitment that no matter
what, I'm not going to abandon myself in the ways I have in the
past. It means that regardless of what is happening outside of me,
regardless of what is happening physically, emotionally, or mentally,
I'm committed to loving and nurturing myself. I'm committed
to spirituality, and I'm not going to let that go regardless of how I
think, feel, or act. I do not neglect or abandon me when the times
get tough. I take care of me today. I am absolute love and power
for myself today. No one else can abandon me. It can feel like
abandonment when someone else leaves, does not show up, or does
not honor a commitment to me; but no rejection from another cuts
as deeply as when I reject and abandon myself. The pain, in fact,
is so deep, so severe, that I numb it out. For that reason it may
feel like the pain others cause me is more intense, when in reality it
is nothing compared to the pain I cause myself when I
abandon and reject me.

*I'm committed to myself today. I love myself today. I am the most
important person in my world today. I take care of me no matter what.
I am committed to me.*

19

RESENTMENT

RELATIONSHIPS

....

"Those who are free of resentful thoughts
surely find peace."
Siddhartha Gautama, the Buddha

Anger is about the present, whereas resentment relates to the past.
It is a re-experiencing of past events and the old feelings of anger
connected to them. Resentment is created when one becomes angry
at a person, institution, or situation, and holds onto that anger.

People can hold onto resentment for many years, refusing to let
go, forgive, or forget, carrying their resentment wherever they go,
weighing themselves down and using up their attention and energy
with it. Over time, the cause of the original anger may be forgotten,
while the resentment remains like smoldering embers that are left
after the flames of a fire have died down. The fire no longer rages,
but the embers remain hot and capable of causing more fires in
the future unless they are extinguished. As long as these embers
continue to burn, they create negative distractions that take time,
attention, and energy away from my pain recovery. I can overcome
resentments by resisting the urge to be a channel for anger or
resentment of others. The anger and resentment directed at others
can be seductive. It can have an almost magnetic pull. I won't buy
into it and resist the urge to join others in their misery.

By focusing on people and situations I'm angry and resentful toward,
I'm out of balance emotionally and typically feeling more pain. I focus
instead on my own recovery and balance.

MAINTAINING BALANCE

PHYSICAL BALANCE

"The world is full of cactus, but we don't have to sit on it."
Will Foley

If I sleep the wrong way and my back is really throbbing, or I twist my shoulder while lifting something heavy, or it is raining and cold, causing my joints to ache—these can cause an acute worsening of my usual painful states and need to be addressed without medication for me to stay in balance.

Unfortunately, there is no warning sign when any of these things may happen. By definition, accidents happen without notice. Bad weather can come "out of the blue" and cause my joints to ache—I can't rely on the weather forecaster every day to warn me about how I'm going to be feeling physically. I go about my day, week, or month, not really thinking about what I'm doing, and then I just lift something the wrong way, and there I go—back into a physical crisis. The point for me is that I always need to be prepared, and can't wait until something happens to expect to be in physical balance. One way I can easily protect myself and my recovery is by making a habit of taking care of my body. I don't have to become a fanatic, but neither do I have to go through life assuming that troubles will never arise. I'm human—my body needs proper care and preventive maintenance to thrive.

I'm making a habit of eating nutritious foods, avoiding toxins, exercising regularly, getting enough sleep, and practicing relaxation, so when a flare-up happens, as it will—I'm prepared.

VICTIM-THINKING

MENTAL BALANCE

···

*"If you think of yourself as a victim, if your mind frame is
one of self-pity, your capacity to experience relief from
chronic pain and stay clean will be greatly diminished."*
Adapted from Pain Recovery: How to Find Balance
and Reduce Suffering from Chronic Pain

A symptom of the disease of addiction is the tendency or, at the
minimum, a capacity to believe in the inherent truth and accuracy
of thoughts. If I work off the assumption that all my thoughts are
fact—that they are all true and valid without examination—
I find myself out of balance and at risk of victim-thinking
that goes unchecked.

Before emotion or action takes place in any situation, a thought
process occurs. There is an initial thought about my pain or
circumstances that results in my victim-thinking. Victim-thinking
is a downward spiral that usually leads to inaction, depression,
anger, resentment, and, consequently, an increased intensity of
pain. Because of my chronic pain I don't have the luxury of victim-
thinking because such thoughts about my pain actually make the
pain worse. When pain strikes, I get to focus on the solution and
think about the actions I'm taking. Then the pain does not
last as long as it once did.

*I am not a victim today. I do not have the luxury of thinking that
I'm a victim, and in the areas of my life where I recognize
victim-thinking, I take action today.*

FEELINGS
EMOTIONAL BALANCE

....

*"Flow with whatever may happen and let
your mind be free. Stay centered by accepting
whatever you are doing. This is the ultimate."*
Zhuangzi

I've learned that emotional balance means that I accept my
emotions and know that it's okay to feel whatever I'm feeling. I'm
more independent of the opinions and beliefs of others and I pay
closer attention to my inner voice and connection to my higher
power than I did before. I identify my feelings and recognize that
my feelings are a major part of me—but not all of me. Noticing and
accepting my feelings is self-acceptance, but self-acceptance is not
an excuse for complacency. To make the changes I desire in my life
I have to accept myself first, then move on.

It takes much less energy to accept my feelings than it takes to fight
and suppress them. Accepting my feelings—especially negative
feelings—helps prevent them from recurring. I'm able to change
them. I shift my energy to productive thoughts and actions when
I accept the way I feel. It frees me to move forward with things I'd
rather be focusing on. Those new thoughts and actions change the
way I feel. The cycle of the four points of balance continues.

*I accept my feelings exactly the way they are today. By accepting
them I shift my energy to productive thoughts and actions, allowing
the feelings to follow.*

COMPASSION

SPIRITUAL BALANCE

"Compassion is easier to see when it occurs
than to describe when it does not...compassion
is not about being or trying to 'make nice.'
It is the attentive, respectful acknowledgment of the
basic humanness of all people, particularly
those who anger, frighten, or harm us."
Of Character: Building Assets in Recovery

Balance requires that I have compassion for others and for myself. I can't say things to myself that I wouldn't say to a small child who was in pain. I show myself that level of love and understanding. I give myself the respect, acknowledgment, and attentiveness that I deserve.

I stay in spiritual balance by showing others and myself the compassion I would show to a small child who was in pain or who was acting up because their needs were not being met.

REACTIONS TO SITUATIONS

RELATIONSHIPS

"The first reaction to truth is hatred."

Tertullian

First reactions are often extreme. It is only upon reflection that we may react with moderation. Life, death of a loved one, illness—my reactions to these universal life experiences are the only things I really have power over. I can laugh about the good times, cry about the bad times, and in recovery I never have to be alone through the hard times. For example, I can let the end of a relationship provide me with motivation to change, hoping that perhaps its ending is the beginning of something even better. Maybe the loss of a job is the best thing that could happen to me because I would have never looked for something better on my own. Whatever the situation, I don't have to let my first reaction be my last today.

I don't have to let my initial reaction to a situation determine my life today. I may find a situation unpleasant, and I may not approve. But today I simply ask my higher power for acceptance. Even if I cannot accept a situation completely at first, I ask my higher power for the willingness to be willing—if that's what it takes. Sometimes acceptance comes slowly, but if I am willing, eventually it comes.

RESPONSIBILITY FOR ACTIONS

PHYSICAL BALANCE

"I develop and execute healthy responses to troublesome thoughts and feelings. I make a habit of taking responsibility for myself by exercising, meditating, getting enough sleep, and eating properly. I work hard, arrive at places on time, participate in social and family activities, and refrain from gossiping because I know that these are all actions I take to take responsibility for my recovery today. Right action for me includes the 'golden rule,' doing unto others as I would have them do unto me. It also includes participating in support groups and giving to others as well as accepting help."

Pain Recovery: How to Find Balance and
Reduce Suffering from Chronic Pain

When my actions are balanced, I'm taking responsibility for my recovery. I take the needed steps to deal with increased pain that may occur from time to time to ensure that I don't need to take opioids, and by so doing take responsibility for the pain that may come up tomorrow.

As the prominent American psychiatrist William James said, "Action may not bring happiness, but there is no happiness without action."

POSITIVE VS. NEGATIVE THOUGHTS

MENTAL BALANCE

"Combine the extremes,
and you will have the true center."
Karl Wilhelm Friedrich Schlegel

One form of extreme thinking is to believe that things are fine
no matter what the reality is. This is often mislabeled as positive
thinking, but it's really a potentially dangerous way of thinking that
flies in the face of reality. This form of positive thinking is
also another form of denial. This is not seeing reality as it is and can
lead to consequences such as underestimating potential problems,
ignoring negative realities, not taking care of myself, and placing
myself in risky situations. It is best to maintain the "true center"
of balance in my thoughts and feelings than to live at the edges,
or at the extremes.

It is okay to have positive thoughts as long as I'm also taking a look
at and acknowledging the realities of my situation. I need to make
sure more than anything that my thinking is followed up by positive
action. Thinking positively about my life—if that life consists
of sitting around all day and watching TV, ignoring all other
responsibilities, and eating unhealthy foods—is not going to help in
my recovery, pay the bills, or replace exercise and hard work.

*I focus on having positive thoughts today; knowing negative thoughts
are a warning sign of imbalance and always lead to imbalance in other
areas of my life. When I'm in balance I am living in pain recovery.*

COMPASSION

EMOTIONAL BALANCE

....

"It is lack of love for ourselves that inhibits our
compassion toward others. If we make friends
with ourselves, then there is no obstacle to opening
our hearts and minds to others."

Unknown

Compassion is usually talked about and thought about in terms of
feeling sympathy, empathy, or love for someone else. What I do not
realize is that through practicing this love and caring for others I am
actually learning how to have that same compassion for myself.

I take it easy on myself. I talk to myself as I would talk to
a newcomer to recovery. I allow myself peace and freedom.
When my head starts to tell me that I should be someone else,
something else, somewhere else, or doing more or less, I stop and
take a moment to reassure myself in a loving way that recovery
is a process and not an event.

*I take the time with myself as I would anyone else whom I care for
deeply. I go out of my way to be loving and kind to me.*

EATING HABITS,
SELF-CARE
PHYSICAL BALANCE

"Self-love, my liege, is not so vile a sin as self-neglecting."
William Shakespeare

What I eat every day has a profound effect on how I feel.
My food plays a major role in my health and well-being.
I remember learning in *Pain Recovery* that the foods I eat
may fight pain in four distinct ways:

 by reducing damage to the site of my injury;

 by working inside my brain to reduce pain sensitivity;

 by acting as painkillers on nerves; and

 by helping my body fight inflammation.

A healthy diet enhances my life and helps me fight many chronic
diseases that often lead to chronic pain or make it worse. Without
a doubt, being and feeling healthy helps me fight pain sensations.

*I pay attention to my eating habits today. I make sure that I am
eating well and know that by eating well I'm helping my body so
that my body can help me.*

FEELINGS OF ISOLATION

RELATIONSHIPS

"Oh, but he was a tight-fisted hand at the grind-stone,
Scrooge! A squeezing, wrenching, grasping, scraping,
clutching, covetous, old sinner! Hard and sharp as flint,
from which no steel had ever struck out generous fire;
secret, and self-contained, and solitary as an oyster."

Charles Dickens

In relationships, sometimes I can feel Scrooge-like—I want to be "secret, and self-contained, and solitary as an oyster." These words describe me well, especially when my chronic pain has me feeling like isolating. Today, when I begin to feel that familiar pull toward isolation, I remember to reach out to another person in recovery, getting out of the house and going to a recovery group meeting, being sociable once I'm there, extending my hand to a newcomer, and praying to my higher power—from whom I can never really be isolated, except, of course, by my own choice.

I've learned in pain recovery that I do not have the "luxury" of isolating myself. I must remember that isolation is the slippery slope back to a life dependent on medication. This doesn't mean I can never be alone or choose to spend time by myself. In fact, some time alone is good for me. Today I understand the difference between isolation and solitude.

When I spend time alone today, it's because I am clear of my intention to be in solitude, spending time for devotion one-on-one with my higher power.

SELF-CARE
PHYSICAL BALANCE

....

"The perfect man of old looked after himself first
before looking to help others."
Chuang Tzu

Learning to care truly starts with learning to care for myself
physically. In pain recovery I learn how to care for myself as
opposed to catering to my pain. I took great care in catering to
my pain when I was in active addiction by continuing to feed and
nurture it. I was singularly focused on giving my pain what
I perceived as its needs.

I centered my entire life around my chronic pain—being
in recovery means shifting that care to my own physical strengths
and well-being. Self-care means centering my life around my pain
recovery. I show real, healthy, loving care for myself by focusing first
on my recovery. I care for myself the way I would a small child who
is sick but does not want to take his or her medicine or does not
want to stay in bed in order to recuperate—I am that child
and today I lovingly make sure I am getting enough sleep, exercise,
and fresh air, eating my vegetables, and resting when
I'm not feeling well.

*I care for myself, nurturing my physical body rather than catering
to it in my pain. I do this by focusing on those things I must do for
my pain recovery, knowing that physical balance requires working
on the things that I can do.*

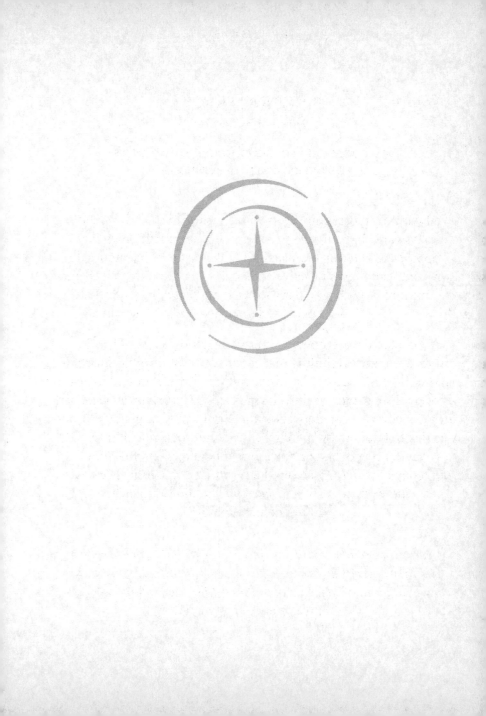

{ OCTOBER }

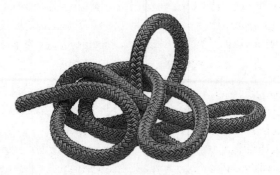

MONITORING AND WARNING SIGNS
MENTAL BALANCE

....

*"He who knows others is wise.
He who knows himself is enlightened."*
Lao Tzu

Just because I'm living drug-free and in pain recovery does not mean that I am always in perfect balance. It is just as important today as it ever was to maintain physical, mental, emotional, and spiritual balance, because I have more to lose today. I need to make sure that I am staying in balance. I ask myself these questions and may be surprised at the responses about my mental balance.

Am I having negative thoughts today? Have I been thinking that I am a victim of someone or something? Do I believe that I have no control of my life? Am I thinking things are worse than they really are? Or am I over-elated? This, too, can be a warning sign of imbalance.

If I answer yes to any of these questions, I need to take action to correct this mental imbalance. Chances are that if I'm imbalanced in this area, it has affected other areas of my recovery. Journaling, prayer, meditation, service, or work with a therapist or sponsor can help me identify and correct the causes of imbalance in my life today.

I talk to my sponsor and pain recovery support group about the areas where I feel mentally imbalanced. I use others as a sounding board for my thoughts, because speaking them aloud often points me toward a solution.

CATASTROPHIZING

EMOTIONAL BALANCE

"Every tomorrow has two handles. We can take hold of
it with the handle of anxiety or the handle of faith."

Henry Ward Beecher

There are two kinds of catastrophizing. One makes mountains out
of molehills, or big problems out of little ones. It's grounded in a
negative viewpoint of actual events—"I'm late for work…I'm going
to get fired…I'll lose my home…I'll be living on the street!" The
other occurs when we look to future events or events that aren't
even likely to happen, and anticipate all the things that are bound
to go wrong—whether or not they have a basis in reality. We then
create a reality around those thoughts—"It's bound to all go wrong
for me." Because we believe something will go wrong, we can
often make it go wrong.

It's important for me to maintain balance between keeping
a rational "lid" on my expectations of events, not letting my hopes
become too high, and thinking everything will turn out for
the worst, or catastrophizing.

*I know the four points of balance are not a miracle cure for what ails
me, but with diligence and persistent effort, balancing the points can
lead to solutions for whatever I'm experiencing, helping me live a more
meaningful and purposeful life.*

COURAGE

SPIRITUAL BALANCE

"Courage is the price life exacts for granting peace."
Amelia Earhart

It takes courage to find spiritual balance. Spiritual balance requires giving up ideas and things that have not worked for me in the past. Letting go is the key element to spiritual connection and the balance within. I cannot be balanced while I hold onto destructive behaviors and addictive behaviors. Changing my behaviors is frightening, but walking through that fear demonstrates courage. By walking through my fear I experience the freedom that is on the other side. I experience what I could not in the past because my mind, body, and spirit were too preoccupied with something that was actually destroying me. When I'm in destructive action I do not leave room for spirituality to enter my life. When I stop the destructive action I'm already in spiritual balance, but it takes time for the feelings to catch up.

Courage is what I have when I step out of the rain, sure that in time the warmth of the sun will dry me. I practice courage, and get to experience what I was seeking all along: love, compassion, acceptance, connection, light, and freedom. I never found those things despite all that I did to get them during my addiction. In letting go, in being courageous in my efforts to allow balance into my life, I realize I had these qualities all along, and that I can share them with others.

I practice courage when I release all that is harmful and destructive in my life, to make room for all that I truly desired when I was trying to manage my own life and my feelings through active addiction.

INVENTORY

RELATIONSHIPS

....

"One of the benefits of being in pain recovery is that I
have enhanced many of the relationships in my life."
Pain Recovery: How to Find Balance and
Reduce Suffering from Chronic Pain

If anything in my relationships needs changing, I understand today
that the most positive changes are often the result of small, slow,
incremental alterations. I have also learned that when something
about a relationship bothers or upsets me, I need to look at my own
part in the problem through the inventory process laid out in the
Twelve Steps; after all, my own part is the only part I can change.

*I'm focusing on my part in relationships today—what I can bring
to them that is positive, as well as what needs to be changed. I don't
point the finger at others; I keep the focus on the one thing I have
power to change: my behavior.*

MANY PATHS OF SPIRITUALITY

PHYSICAL BALANCE

"There are no drawbacks to seeking
a spiritual experience. You have nothing to lose
and everything to gain. All that is required is
for you to be open-minded and willing."

Pain Recovery: How to Find Balance and
Reduce Suffering from Chronic Pain

People may share their beliefs with me, and it may feel like
they're trying to preach, but I remember that I'm free to choose
what I believe today. I don't judge others for their beliefs; I just
keep doing what works for me, monitoring my progress as I move
forward, applying what works and leaving the rest. I write, read,
develop a support group through meetings, work the steps, exercise,
pray, meditate, share, be of service, stay in the moment, clear
resentments and unresolved feelings, laugh, cry, express gratitude,
accept my pain, cherish opportunity, and make progress toward
balance. All of these are paths, ways, and means to spirituality;
not one of them is denominational, religious, dogmatic, or
specifically defined. Every single one of these paths leads to
health and healing. I work on as many as I can. Spirituality
is the light and fire inside me that believes, holds onto the idea
that I can rise above the circumstances of my life, and knows
that I can be better and do better.

*I work on each aspect of my program, knowing that each one is an
aspect of spirituality, a path to healing and recovery.*

SPIRITUAL AWAKENING

MENTAL BALANCE

"No human being ever learns to live until he has awakened to the dormant power within him."
William James

A spiritual awakening is sometimes just a state of mind. Something as simple as a different perspective can be a spiritual awakening for someone like me, who was trapped in believing there was only one way: the abuse of medication. The chronic focus on an irremediable pain and the insanity of believing there is some thing, pill, person, place, idea, etc., that could change the way I feel is always going to be a part of me. That's a painful acceptance, especially when struggling during the withdrawal that can last weeks, or even months. But even during the withdrawal period I can start to have a clearer mind, see things a little differently, get moments of gratitude, hope, belief, faith, trust, acceptance, and— possibly—joy. I have hope that maybe recovery *is* possible. With that in my heart I send a message back to my mind that is focused and changed, thinking instinctively of ways to protect myself. Recovery is the healing and protection I need today.

As I awaken, refreshed and renewed, I release myself from yesterday's pain as if from a bad dream. A new day awaits me, and I am ready.

AMENDS

EMOTIONAL BALANCE

....

*"Gladly we desire to make other men perfect,
but we will not amend our own fault."*
Thomas à Kempis

I have learned from looking at the four points of balance in my life that in order to live my amends to my friends and family, I must be there for myself first. My emotional needs and wants must be tended to or I am left vulnerable to having my pain take hold and regain control. By tending to myself first I am actually making amends to others in my life, even when it doesn't feel that way. I take care of my recovery and become able to make my amends to those around me.

I put my recovery first. Though this may sound selfish, actually it is not. Once I have taken care of myself the amends to others follow naturally, but this is not possible otherwise.

IMPATIENCE

SPIRITUAL BALANCE

....

*"The two most powerful warriors
are patience and time."*

Leo Nikolaevich Tolstoy

The door to my inner self is a door that opens out, but my
impatience is a force that is always leaning on it, trying vainly to
push it in. I wonder why it doesn't open. So I lean on it harder. I
start banging on the door and pushing, trying every way I can to
force the door to open inward. All I need to do is step back and
pull. When I'm acting impatiently there is no room for stepping
back. There is no room for allowance or tolerance. When this
happens, I can realize that I am actually what is standing in the way
of achieving my own desires. When I step out of the way, I make
room for that connection with my recovery to take place. Instead
of leaning on the door I want to enter, I wander down the hall,
going through other doors—meetings, recovery, sponsors, steps,
pain recovery maintenance—and while I'm focused on those
other things, the door to my soul opens and I'm standing
in the doorway before I even notice.

*Rather than leaning on a door that opens out, I make room today
for that door to open by working on other things. I wait patiently by
practicing pain recovery as the objects of my desires come to me.*

RELATIONSHIP PATTERNS

RELATIONSHIPS

....

"It is important to take inventory of my current
relationships so that I can identify those that help
or hinder my quest for balance. I assess my relationships
and alter or let go of unhealthy associations and
focus on healthy relationships with people who
are sincerely interested in my well-being."
Adapted from Pain Recovery: How to Find Balance
and Reduce Suffering from Chronic Pain

Relationship patterns are established early in life. Our
parents, role models, friends, etc., influence the way we view
ourselves and others, and have an emotional impact throughout
our lives. If I don't examine these patterns I'll tend to repeat them,
whether they are healthy or unhealthy. Identifying my own patterns
is a significant step in helping me to choose relationships in which
I support others and they support me in a mutually beneficial
give-and-take.

*I take inventory of the relationships in my life and pay attention
to those that are not mutual and are not helping me in my recovery.
I work with my sponsor, counselor, or therapist in determining that
it is time to move on.*

MEMORY

PHYSICAL BALANCE

....

"My ability to get through a day living with my pain
has given me strength. Since chronic pain frequently
cannot be seen or measured, unlike acute pain,
doctors, colleagues, friends, or family may question
or doubt your pain. In effect, it doesn't matter if anyone
believes you, but it is extremely important for you
to acknowledge that all pain is real."
Pain Recovery: How to Find Balance and
Reduce Suffering from Chronic Pain

During the course of my pain recovery there may be times when
it's easy to feel like I'm "recovered," but I must remember that
recovery is a lifelong process. No matter how long I have been
practicing the principles of recovery and living with my pain
without the use of medication, I must always remember and
acknowledge that I do have chronic pain. I must keep this fresh
in my memory. Addiction could take control of my life again at
any moment, so I must stay vigilant in my recovery.

*I take a moment to acknowledge my pain and the power it has
had over my life. I remember where I have been, and take note of
where I am now and where I am heading in recovery.*

SELF-TALK, SELF-CARE

MENTAL BALANCE

"While you may be powerless over the self-talk that first enters your mind, you are not powerless over what you do in response to it. You can detach from your thoughts— observe them, question their accuracy, dispute or talk back to them, and, ultimately, change them."

Pain Recovery: How to Find Balance and
Reduce Suffering from Chronic Pain

The way that I talk to myself is part of how I take care of myself today. I identify automatic thoughts and self-talk about my chronic pain. I took a look at what is true and what is not. I also realize that as a result of my thoughts and self-talk in the past, I made decisions to follow pathways that ended up making my pain worse. I need to keep fresh in my memory exactly what following these paths led to.

I begin to change by talking to myself the way I would to another person who was recovering or just beginning to kick painkillers. What would I say to that person if he was complaining about his pain? What would I tell him if he wanted to give up? Or if she were saying any of the things that I say to myself during any given day, how would I respond? Would my words be kind or harsh? Would my tone be loving or cruel? Often, I say things to myself that I wouldn't say to my worst enemy. I do not allow that kind of self-talk to just go unchecked today. My self-talk today is kind and encouraging.

I talk to myself the way I would to a person who is just beginning the pain recovery process. Many of my actions start with thoughts; those thoughts start with self-talk. Today I make sure my self-talk is healthy and supportive of my recovery.

ADVERSITY

EMOTIONAL BALANCE

....

"Adversity has the effect of eliciting talents, which in prosperous circumstances would have lain dormant."
Horace

When I'm going through challenging times with my pain, I start to question my ability to get through it without the use of medications. In my mind I know the right thing to do, but my emotions start to get out of whack and things get blown out of proportion. My pain flares up, and it makes me feel depressed or anxious. My emotional reaction to the adversity I'm facing has a direct effect on my ability to tolerate my pain. When I become emotionally charged in challenging situations, it puts my physical body at risk, and then my recovery is in jeopardy.

During these times it is more important than ever to stay close and connected to people in my support group. I communicate my emotional difficulty to them and listen to their experiences in similar situations. More than that, I know that I am not alone, and there is nothing that I can't get through in pain recovery without using medications or acting on old behaviors.

I look at emotional adversity as an opportunity for growth. I renew my commitment to recovery.

CATASTROPHIZING

SPIRITUAL BALANCE

....

"Some of us have a tendency to get caught
up in spinning elaborate scenarios related to events
that may never actually occur, and spend considerable
time and emotional energy looking for potential
trouble, as well as for solutions to problems that don't
exist. For instance, I sense pain in a specific area of my
body that may be uncomfortable, but in and of itself
is not that big a deal. However, my self-talk tells me,
'This is horrible! It's going to spread to my entire body.
I'll be in intense pain and have to spend the day,
maybe even several days, in bed!'"
*Pain Recovery: How to Find Balance and
Reduce Suffering from Chronic Pain*

Thinking that catastrophe is inevitable has considerable influence
on my experience of pain and my perceived options. The first step
in interrupting this process is to become aware of it and realize what
I'm thinking. Only then can I make an informed decision about
how I want to proceed, based on the options available.

*I can think differently about something I would have considered a
catastrophe before, in order to regain/maintain balance in my life.*

FELLOWSHIP

RELATIONSHIPS

....

"Gratitude preserves old friendships, and procures new."
Unknown

I was taken aback the first time I heard a member share at a
meeting of my recovery fellowship that they were "grateful" to be an
addict. "Grateful?" I had to think about that for a little while, and
ask my sponsor and other fellowship friends what a person in our
fellowship, considering all we'd been through, could mean by that.
Today I have come to understand that I have much to be grateful
for—the fellowship itself, for one thing.

Before entering pain recovery, I was alone with my problems. And
the more I tried to solve my problems by myself, the worse they
seemed to become. My solutions turned out to be no solutions
at all, yet when I was left to my own devices, they were the best I
could do. In my recovery fellowship today, I have scores of friends
who offer help when asked. They are always ready to lend a hand or
an ear. I'm sure to find others in my fellowship who have shared the
same problems as I have, and who can show me by their example
how they overcame the problems in their own lives.

Today I can say that I'm grateful to be an addict in recovery,
a member in good standing of my recovery fellowship.

*Reaching out is not just about getting my needs met, but about
finding groups such as twelve-step meetings as places to find others who
can help me and who also need the help that I can provide because
of my own experiences.*

OCTOBER

15

RECOVERY

PHYSICAL BALANCE

*"To change one's life: Start immediately.
Do it flamboyantly."*
William James

Before recovery, I was completely identified with my pain. My entire life was consumed with being in pain. There was no one in my life who did not know that I was in pain because most of the time it was my excuse for not going to work, partaking in activities, or taking care of my responsibilities. It was all I talked about, seemingly. I had to change.

Today I am in recovery, and that's how I want to be identified—not as a person in chronic pain. I am taking care of my chronic pain and my recovery. When people see me, I want them to think first of my recovery and not of my pain. While my pain is always a *part* of me, my pain is not me. My life is rich today. It includes many different things, and the focus of my life is not on addiction or suffering, but on exercising, meditation, study, recovery, family, and friends. I have much to talk about, and I talk about those areas of my life I want to feed, nurture, and be identified with.

*When someone asks me about my pain, I change the focus
and answer them by talking about something that I would rather
be identified with—my recovery, my activities, and what I am
doing with my life today.*

PATIENCE

MENTAL BALANCE

....

"I'm actively and patiently changing my thought
patterns; however, my thoughts remain consistent
in the belief that if I apply the techniques and practice
the skills learned in pain recovery, my recovery, and
my thinking, will stay balanced. I understand that the
most effective way to acquire new skills or to get better
at anything is to learn the techniques that work and
practice them relentlessly."
*Pain Recovery: How to Find Balance and
Reduce Suffering from Chronic Pain*

When I start to think that I should be further along or in better
condition, I think about any sport or activity that must be learned. If
I am to excel at anything I have to practice, and I must be patient as
I learn this new skill. It does not come overnight. But success more
than anything is a state of mind. I must think of myself as a success
and then trust in the process of pain recovery and the techniques
I'm learning as I patiently practice my program of recovery.

*I am patient with myself and understand that changing thought
patterns does not happen easily or quickly, but comes slowly over time.*

ACTIONS

EMOTIONAL BALANCE

....

"Most of us try to 'think our way into good acting.'
Twelve-step recovery recommends that you
'act your way into good thinking.'"
Pain Recovery: How to Find Balance and
Reduce Suffering from Chronic Pain

When I'm in too much pain I can't think straight, and I start
acting on my emotions rather than on my recovery and what is best
for me. I need to monitor and acknowledge my emotions, but at the
same time, the actions I take in my recovery cannot be emotionally
based. I need to pay attention to my emotional reactions to things
and make sure my actions are based on what I know is good
for my recovery.

Pausing, reflecting, and then taking appropriate, loving, recovery-
based action—rather than reacting to situations emotionally—
is what helps me deal with my pain today.

*I try to take actions that are not emotionally charged. I respond
to situations, including my pain, with recovery and the tools and
principles I have acquired in my recovery program.*

ATTITUDE

SPIRITUAL BALANCE

....

*"Could we change our attitude, we should not only see
life differently, but life itself would come to be different.
Life would undergo a change of appearance because
we ourselves had undergone a change in attitude."*
Katherine Mansfield

Attitude can be thought of as the way that I move toward or away
from a situation. What exactly is my attitude toward pain? Do I flee
from my pain like a ship at sea trying to outrun a storm? Do I fight
the pain and increase tension in my body? Pain recovery provides
me with the opportunity to exist between these two extremes and to
work toward achieving balance in all areas of my life. My attitude
is not shaped by the events taking place in my life. My attitude is
shaped by my reaction to events taking place in my life in direct
proportion to my state of imbalance. Attitudes can change.
My attitudes must change if my pain recovery is to be a success.
How my attitude changes is an important aspect of my new
life in pain recovery.

*I use the tools I have been given in recovery to improve my attitude
and to lead a more balanced life. I no longer feel comfortable existing
in the extremes, and instead strive to remain centered and balanced.
My attitude is one of gratitude.*

SEXUALITY

RELATIONSHIPS

> "Chronic pain can interfere with
> a healthy sex life in a number of ways."
> Pain Recovery: How to Find Balance and
> Reduce Suffering from Chronic Pain

Since chronic pain entered my life, my sex life has changed. I may have difficulty being/feeling sexual, perhaps because my self-esteem has diminished and I feel less attractive to a partner, or less able to perform. Changing roles or household patterns because of chronic pain may also have affected my sexuality. I find I may anticipate or fear increased pain as a result of sexual activity, which can further interfere with my performance, or cause me to avoid sex altogether. I may also have decreased sexual function because of my past drug use. Prescribed medications, even when not used abusively, can have a dampening effect on my libido. These reactions are commonplace; I am not unique.

There is no need for me to be ashamed or to renounce a sex life altogether. If these issues affect me I can talk to my doctor, counselor, sponsor, and sexual partner today. These discussions allow me to be honest, which creates intimacy with my partner.

When I'm at home I keep a pain journal for jotting down points and reflecting on occasions when I am intimate with my partner. I note at what points my pain occurred, and what I was doing when the pain subsided. I discuss these issues with my doctor, counselor, sponsor, and partner. I am a sexual being, even with chronic pain. I give and receive pleasure today.

OPENNESS, WILLINGNESS, TENACITY

PHYSICAL BALANCE

....

"Where the willingness is great,
the difficulties cannot be great."
Niccolò Machiavelli

The work I've done in pain recovery has helped me notice my pain in very different ways. I'm open to the changing experience and am amazed at how different my pain feels today. Techniques I've learned in pain recovery, through the *Pain Recovery* workbook, attending pain support groups, physical therapies, counseling, and twelve-step work have helped. Some techniques have worked more than others. How much each technique helps depends a lot on how much openness, willingness, and tenacity I have.

I have to be patient with the process of recovery, using the tools I've learned along the way, and I know I cannot expect results overnight. I continue to be open to the tools I've learned, to be willing to try new ones, and to have the tenacity to continue with a certain technique until I have seen how it works. I cannot expect results overnight. I need to practice tenacity by continuing to work with my counselor or sponsor. I remind myself that pain recovery takes time.

I remember that the techniques I learn in pain recovery work to the extent that I work them. A great deal of my recovery depends on my openness, willingness, and tenacity.

THE PLASTIC BRAIN
MENTAL BALANCE

....

"Scientists have learned that the human brain is plastic—
not plastic like a picnic coffee spoon or a CD cover,
but plastic in that it can change, both physically and
functionally. Every day, the brain adapts and compensates
in response to the right stimulus. Connections can be
rewired and/or refined; the brain's gray matter can
thicken, and new neurons can be produced."
A Day without Pain

It's a blessing knowing I can mold my plastic brain into whatever I
want, as long as I put the work into it. It's quick and easy to change
my brain with the instant chemicals that are manufactured by
multibillion-dollar pharmaceutical companies and genetically
engineered to tip the scales of balance in my brain artificially.
However, nothing is more powerful than nature. The way in which
I can change my own brain naturally takes more time and effort,
but it is more powerful than any drug, including the drug alcohol,
that I can ingest. In recovery, I've learned I can change my brain
by going to a meeting, calling my sponsor, or talking with another
person in recovery. I can do yoga or practice prayer and meditation.
These ways in which I change my brain may take time, but the
memory built from slow and sustained growth is far more
powerful than artificial alteration.

*I can change my brain to be the way I want it. I work daily on molding
and exercising the muscle of my brain using the healthy tools of
recovery instead of looking to the quick fix of chemicals.*

OPEN-MINDEDNESS
EMOTIONAL BALANCE

....

"People often confuse being open-minded
with not having a firm position. In fact, having firm
convictions, based on criteria we have decided are
important to us, is almost a requirement of being
open-minded. Being open-minded means listening
attentively and respectfully to the position of another.
It does not require we fully understand, agree,
or support the position."
Of Character: Building Assets in Recovery

I can have an intense emotional reaction to people in my life.
In fact, the longer I stay in recovery and the more in touch with my
own emotions I get, the more intense my reactions can become.
But this does not stop me from having an open mind. In pain
recovery, I learn to practice principles even when I'm feeling
intense feelings and reactions. Actually, recovery is about practicing
those principles *especially* when I'm in a pain spike or
in a heightened emotional state. Emotional maturity is being able
to feel my feelings, and at the same time, respect someone else.
I can listen to another, feel more than one feeling at a time,
and practice principles.

*Because I stand for recovery and believe in the four points of balance,
I listen to other points of view. When I'm feeling contrary or belligerent,
I realize I can have my feelings and an open mind at the same time.
They are not mutually exclusive. I get to have more than one feeling
at a time today and do more than one thing simultaneously.*

APPRECIATION

SPIRITUAL BALANCE

....

*"The deepest principle in human nature
is the craving to be appreciated."*
William James

Many doctors, therapists, and others professionals have tried, and continue to try, to help me deal with my pain. No matter how good they may be at what they do, they do not feel my pain. Many have not had the firsthand experience of chronic pain. I must accept this fact and appreciate their efforts to help me even though they do not fully understand. I look to the fellowship in my twelve-step program and my support group for identification. It is through that identification with others who have actually experienced and continue to experience pain like mine that I find comfort during my time of need. The professionals I work with can and often do empathize and sympathize with me for the pain I am experiencing, but it is with my fellows in pain recovery that I truly experience identification.

As part of my acceptance of my pain, I avoid the urge to resent those who are not in pain. I appreciate their efforts to comfort me and strive to show my appreciation for those efforts.

I thank those who comfort me and help me to deal with my pain. I do so daily and hope to brighten their day by showing my appreciation.

FOUR POINTS OF BALANCE

RELATIONSHIPS

....

"Be courteous to all but intimate with few,
and let those few be well tried before
you give them your confidence."
George Washington

I recognize that the more balanced I am, the better my relationships are. I also know that the more emotionally healthy I am, the healthier the people I will attract. Today, I choose to be in relationships that support and nurture me without unleashing any codependence or enabling, whether mine or my partner's. As a result, today I have people in my life who lovingly tell me the truth because they put my well-being above their own fear of my reaction. I ask for help whenever I need it, knowing it is a sign of strength, not weakness. I maintain my own health, and in so doing have healthy people in my life whom I can count on to help me in my recovery. If I see that I am attracting unhealthy people into my life who are not coming to me to change for the better, but instead are coming to me to commiserate, or to be codependent or enabled, I take a look at my own health and why I'm attracting those types of people into my life today. I make changes with the help of my sponsor and healthy program friends.

I focus on my own health and well-being, and in so doing attract healthy people into my life who tell me the truth and support me in my choice to remain in pain recovery.

MOVEMENT
PHYSICAL BALANCE

....

"Regular and sustained physical activity is
beneficial to virtually every system in the body.
During exercise your body releases chemicals
called endorphins, which naturally relieve pain
and also help to lessen anxiety and depression."

*Pain Recovery: How to Find Balance and
Reduce Suffering from Chronic Pain*

I need to pay attention to all areas of my life and make sure that I
am in balance. Have I exercised today? Am I eating healthy foods?
Am I increasing my physical abilities regularly and gaining more
function, or am I losing function? How is my sleep? How is my sex
life? Do I work and support my family to the extent that I am able?

As part of regular maintenance in my recovery, I need to continue
to ask myself these questions. There may be certain areas of my
recovery that need more attention than others. These are often
the areas I tend to neglect, but I remind myself to attend to all
my physical needs—not just the ones that are easy or fun. That's
the way to improve my function.

*I pay attention to the physical balance I have (or do not have)
in my life. I take a physical balance inventory, noting the areas
that need more attention, in order to keep a healthy balance
in my pain recovery program.*

COURAGE

MENTAL BALANCE

....

"Being in recovery is about becoming consciously aware
of self-destructive and self-defeating thoughts and
behaviors and replacing those behaviors with healthy,
growth-enhancing ways of relating to oneself, others,
and to the world. As a result, recovery takes strength and
courage to pursue and to maintain on a daily basis."
Of Character: Building Assets in Recovery

It's not easy to take a look at my thoughts and behaviors, especially
when I'm in pain. Sometimes I fear that examining my thoughts and
behaviors might increase my pain. Sometimes it does. The darkest
hour is before dawn. I must remember that the pain of remaining
stuck where I am is greater than the pain of changing. It takes
courage to face the things that have caused me pain. Emotional pain
and mental anguish have only increased my physical pain. To be free
from abusing pain medication, to live with chronic pain, requires
facing those things. Courage means that even though I'm afraid and
don't want to hurt anymore, I do what needs to be done. I make a
habit of monitoring my behaviors and thoughts. I do this through
the use of twelve-step principles, doing my own inventory, being
accountable to a sponsor and support system, attending meetings,
and praying and meditating. I make a habit of acting courageously.

*Courage needs assistance. Courage is action. I make a habit of
acting in courage. I make a habit of acting in steps, sponsorship,
meetings, abstinence, and refraining from old or questionable
behavior. I practice courage today.*

TRUST

EMOTIONAL BALANCE

....

"Wise men put their trust in ideas
and not in circumstances."
Ralph Waldo Emerson

It takes time to trust my feelings, to trust that my response to a situation just might be appropriate to the situation. In the past, and in active addiction, the reaction, the emotion, was completely out of proportion to the situation. The emotion was heightened by unresolved issues, current pain, and fighting the pain. I took it out on everyone. So I got into recovery and almost immediately become *afraid* of my feelings, afraid to trust them, because as I continue to work a recovery program, I see the full effects that my pain has had on me and those around me.

But through working a program I begin to trust my own feelings. I also trust that I won't react to my feelings right away, that I can trust the process of recovery, and I won't just fly off the handle, snap at someone, or make some rash decision based on my feelings on a given day. I trust myself to know that my feelings are not fact.

*Through working a pain recovery program I learn to trust my emotions,
but even while I trust them, I know that everything I do is filtered
through a specific thought process and through an application
of the twelve-step principles.*

INTELLIGENCE
MENTAL BALANCE

"Many difficulties which nature throws in our way may
be smoothed away by the exercise of intelligence."
Titus Livius

I like to think of myself as an intelligent person who thinks clearly,
yet it's true that my trusty thinking once told me it would be a
good idea to abuse my pain medications and look where that got
me! This flawed logic (a product of my strange thinking itself)
was pointed out to me by my sponsor early in pain recovery when
I expressed my difficulty trusting in the wisdom of my newly
discovered higher power.

I still wanted to rely on my own thinking to help me in recovery;
I thought I could judge which of the tools of recovery—meeting
attendance, journaling, step and service work, etc.—I needed and
which I could neglect. Needless to say, until I started accepting
that my own thinking could usually only be trusted to lead me into
trouble, and instead started trusting in my higher power and the
advice, born of experience, of those in my recovery fellowship, I
struggled in recovery. Today my intelligence tells me to trust the
tools of my recovery program instead of acting impulsively; the
results are usually much better.

*I trust the process of recovery, and today I trust my higher power. I use
my intelligence to apply myself to the program of recovery, and I have
no need to ponder or worry about my pain recovery as long as I follow
the simple steps my program outlines so clearly for me.*

INTIMACY

RELATIONSHIPS

"A friend is a person with whom I may be sincere.
Before him I may think aloud."
Ralph Waldo Emerson

Today I am never ashamed to share my most intimate feelings with another in recovery. I reach out to my sponsor, therapist, or closest friends in my fellowship. I can tell them all my fears and doubts, and know that they will listen with sincere understanding. By reaching out I am able to grow in my recovery. This reaching out and sharing is the basis of true intimacy.

My pain recovery support group and my sponsor, therapist, or counselor are available to help me deal with the challenges I face in pain recovery. I understand that by reaching out I am also able to help them in their time of need. I resist the urge to go it alone. I understand this is contrary to my desire to isolate and to feel sorry for myself. I know that by connecting with others who share in my fear, shame, frustration, and anger, all things are possible.

I go to a meeting, call my sponsor, and call someone else in pain recovery. By reaching out and making contact, I fulfill a promise to myself to have a positive day.

COMPASSION
SPIRITUAL BALANCE

"When we behave compassionately to those
expecting anger or retaliation, we disturb their view of
the world and of us in a way that may promote growth
and encourage human connection."
Of Character: Building Assets in Recovery

When I change my behavior in regard to my pain, I disrupt and
disturb the process through which I normally handle the pain.
When I respond to the pain with compassion, I change the way
the signals work in my brain and my body, and essentially can
change the pain itself. Compassion is a powerful tool for me in
pain recovery. It actually has the ability to change the pain itself, to
change the situation, and to change my life. I shake up my view of
my pain, my thought process toward it, and in doing so I promote
my own growth and encourage a spiritual connectedness within me
that is the antidote above all others to the toxic downward spiral that
was killing me or making me a victim of chronic pain. Through
compassion for others and myself, including the way I experience
my chronic pain, I've found a means for living a happy,
joyful, productive life.

*I behave compassionately and shake up my own world and my way
of thinking about my chronic pain, thereby promoting growth and
encouraging connection within myself and with those around me.*

VICTIM-THINKING

MENTAL BALANCE

....

"I can easily forget that I'm in control of my life and return to feeling like a victim of my chronic pain. I may start asking myself again why this has happened to me, what I did to deserve this, etc. However, one of the gifts of pain recovery has been freedom from victim-thinking. This comes about over time, but it does come.

Adapted from Pain Recovery: How to Find Balance and Reduce Suffering from Chronic Pain

Focusing on my pain only keeps me trapped in an endless cycle of victim-thinking—"Why me?" gets me nowhere. My thoughts will try to tell me otherwise, but the antidote to victim-thinking is action, and in my pain recovery program there is plenty of healthy action to take. Meetings, reading, prayer, work with a sponsor or therapist, helping another—all these are the time-tested ways to get me out of my victim-thinking and into recovery.

The way I think influences the way I feel, which in turn affects my actions. I review my action plan for when I turn to negative thoughts: What actions do I take when my thinking turns to that of being a victim? I make sure I have a plan to fight victim-thinking with positive thoughts and actions.

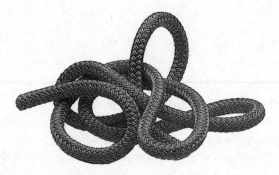

1

WILLINGNESS
EMOTIONAL BALANCE

"Though the strength is lacking,
the willingness is commendable."
Ovid

When I'm feeling good, it's easy to have the willingness to take the actions necessary to do what needs to be done in my life. But then the pain hits. The first thing to get out of balance after my physical pain is my emotional state. My feelings come as a direct result of my level of pain, bypassing the thinking processes, bypassing what I know in recovery. My immediate desire is to fix the pain. When I cannot use drugs, I look to other sources to fix that pain. These other sources may result in my acting out toward my family, not doing what I need to do for my body, wallowing in my pain, or thinking that I can make my pain someone else's problem. When I'm in pain my emotions are the same: loneliness, anger, resentment, fear, shame, guilt, etc.

It is during these heightened states of emotional turmoil that willingness is more important than ever. I demonstrate my willingness; I act on recovery principles rather than acting as my disease tells me to. I wait it out. If there is something I just absolutely need to say or do, I show willingness to be in the recovery process by waiting until the emotional crisis and the increased pain level have passed. Then I can filter everything I say and do through my pain recovery program, not through my pain.

I show willingness, especially when I'm emotionally charged, by practicing restraint instead of just lashing out or doing what I want to do. I "wait it out," regroup, and demonstrate willingness to recover.

ADVERSITY
SPIRITUAL BALANCE

"In adversity, remember to keep an even mind."
Horace

Maintaining balance, while coping with a problem, is the hardest thing for me to do in recovery. When I am feeling exceptional amounts of pain on any given day, it is hard for me to remember that balance is the key to the adversity I face regarding my physical wellness. This balance is what helps me maintain a spiritual outlook on my life and helps me put any problems into perspective.

When I am faced with challenges, physical or otherwise, I remember that the solution in my life is always spiritual in nature. Spirituality requires balance in my life, and that balance requires feeding those areas of my life that I want to grow.

I feed the positive and healthy parts of my life, especially when other parts of my life are causing me turmoil, pain, or discomfort. It is always important for me to focus on all the different areas of my life and recovery.

SLOW, INCREMENTAL CHANGES

RELATIONSHIPS

"Perhaps time's definition of coal is the diamond."
Kahlil Gibran

"We need to talk." Those four little words, when spoken by one partner in a relationship, often translate to "There's something about *you* that I want to change." A more honest way to address the need for change in a relationship when it arises is to take inventory of the situation and work on the only thing I *can* change — me!

I resist the urge to "work on" my relationships, and keep the focus on myself. As I work on my recovery, my relationships become more balanced. The best way for me to resolve relationship issues is through slow, incremental changes based on my desire to achieve balance. This takes time and effort, but so does everything worthwhile. Although it may sound selfish, now is the time for me to receive what I need. Even after time in recovery, I still need to stay focused on receiving what I need and focus on my own recovery rather than the relationship itself. The solution is in the steps and in working on my recovery.

I focus on my recovery and trust that, in so doing, my relationships benefit from that work.

PHYSICAL ABILITIES

PHYSICAL BALANCE

"Use it or lose it."
Unknown

It doesn't matter how young, healthy, or vibrant I am; I need to always work on increasing my physical abilities. Even those in the best shape who work out at the gym daily work on increasing their physical capacities. With chronic pain it's even more important for me to regularly work on increasing my physical abilities.

I am opioid-free and living with my pain, but recovery is an ongoing process that continues forever—even if the pain magically goes away. Part of my recovery is continuing to increase not just my mental, emotional, and spiritual capacity, but my physical capacity as well. Maybe I can walk an extra few minutes. Maybe I can work out a muscle—even just lightly—that I was afraid to work out at all before. Maybe I can get into that yoga posture today. Whatever it may be, I can take safe, simple steps to increase my physical ability and know that by doing so, I am strengthening my body and my recovery.

I have many options available to me to work on physical balance: walking, running, yoga, lifting weights, stretching, swimming, etc. I do something for my body today to work on increasing my physical abilities.

FOCUS ON THE SOLUTION

MENTAL BALANCE

"All pain is real...despite there no longer being an obvious acute physical reason for its presence. In many who have chronic pain, there is not always a concrete and obvious reason for its existence."

A Day without Pain

It's all too easy, even in recovery, to start to question why I have pain or to get into the downward spiral of shame, thinking about what I might have done to cause the pain, what I could have done differently, etc. But that is a backward and unproductive way of thinking about my pain. The reality is that regardless of why or how, my pain is real. It is a part of my life and something I must live with—one day at a time. The only question that I can really ask myself is: "What quality do I want that life to have?"

Recovery is not about getting to the root or reason for the existence of the pain, but continuing a daily practice of my focus on the solution and recovery. It is still the silent and sometimes unnoticed aspect of that life that no one can see or understand, but that needs me to know and accept that it is real. Just as real as the pain is, so is the recovery I have today.

My pain is real today. I do not need to convince anyone, nor does it matter what it is or how or from where it came; what matters is that I'm in recovery and focused on the solution.

IMPATIENCE
EMOTIONAL BALANCE

....

"Have patience with all things,
but chiefly have patience with yourself.
Do not lose courage in considering your own
imperfections, but instantly set about remedying
them—every day begin the task anew."
St. Francis de Sales

In pain recovery, I learn to be patient with myself and my feelings.
Grieving the loss of my old "friends," pain medications and the
lifestyle that accompanied their use, can bring on a whole new kind
of pain. Though they were ultimately bad for me and had to go, it's
natural to feel grief at their loss. These feelings can last a while, and
what's more, they can resurface even when I'm doing everything
that I'm "supposed" to be doing in my recovery. It can be so hard
to stay the course. I get to learn to have patience with my feelings
these days. I get to learn compassion and understanding. I give
myself time to shed a tear and even grieve, but I don't beat myself
up for it. I don't wallow in the feelings of grief. Most importantly,
I don't rebuke myself or get impatient with myself when
I'm having these feelings.

*I am patient with my feelings (emotions), understanding
that my thoughts and actions may be in balance, but that feelings
take time to catch up. I understand and have compassion for myself
and those feelings, knowing that moving through them, experiencing
them, is a lifelong process that I'm learning how to do in a healthy
way in pain recovery.*

CRISIS OF FAITH

SPIRITUAL BALANCE

"Doubt is a pain too lonely
to know that faith is his twin brother."
Kahlil Gibran

Nothing feels more serious to a person in recovery than
of faith. Feeling alienated from my own internal beliefs is p
the most disconcerting thing I've had to experience in reco
I don't like it when I feel doubts about my higher power's lo
or when I feel that I don't know what is right or wrong for my o
spirit. However, learning how to deal with these doubts is a sigi.
of maturity in recovery. I learn how to deal with doubt and pain,
and when I break through to the other side I find great spiritual
growth. I've learned that doubt is not the enemy of faith;
it is an element of faith.

By learning how to walk through to the other side of my own
internal struggles I have strengthened the relationship between my
higher power and myself. I work through the internal adversity in
my recovery by continuing to exercise, meditate, write, and work
my recovery program. It is from these struggles—when no one
outside of myself is telling me I need to do anything—that my
greatest personal accomplishments stem.

*When I feel more fear than faith and want to give up on my recovery
practices, I remind myself that these are often the experiences that lead
to great spiritual growth. I talk to a sponsor, counselor, or fellowship
member about my fears—and I don't give up on my program or myself.*

FINDING MUTUAL
SUPPORT AND ALLIES

RELATIONSHIPS

"Trouble shared is trouble halved."
Scottish proverb

didn't come into this world alone; no human did. That fact alone should tell me that we humans are social animals—we need one another. The first word of the steps of my recovery fellowship tells me that, too. "We" can recover together. There's no "I" in recovery.

I make an effort to reach out to people, one way or another, knowing that having a social network and contact with other people is proven to help me in pain recovery.

SLEEPING

PHYSICAL BALANCE

"We are such stuff as dreams are made of
and our little life is rounded with sleep."
William Shakespeare

Sleep—too much or not enough—is a problem for many people,
not just those with chronic pain.

For many of us in pain recovery it may be tempting to look for easy,
chemical solutions to the problem of sleeplessness, but that's not
an option if I want to maintain my recovery. I work on my sleep
function by making sure that I'm doing a Tenth Step—taking my
personal inventory on a regular basis and making amends where
I need to; praying and meditating; eating right and exercising.
Granted, all these things may not help me perfectly, and in
such cases I reach out to my support group, physical therapist,
acupuncturist, or nutritionist for their help in getting more regular
and sound sleep at night.

On the other end of the spectrum is sleeping too much. In that
case, I need to figure out what function too much sleep might be
fulfilling. If it's just that I'm physically exhausted, that's one thing.
But if I'm using sleep to avoid showing up for life, then that is
something else I may need to look at.

As in all aspects of my recovery, balance is the key.

*I make sure I am monitoring my sleep, and I take the action
necessary to correct what needs to be corrected.*

MEMORY

MENTAL BALANCE

"Brain imaging studies reported by National Institute
of Drug Abuse (NIDA) show that addicted individuals
have physical changes in areas of the brain critical
to judgment, decision making, learning, memory,
and behavior control."
A Day without Pain

It's just a fact of life that my memory has been affected not only by
my chronic pain, but also by my former active drug addiction. My
memory may or may not come back over time, so I need to take this
into consideration in recovery. It's important for me to write things
down, particularly my medical appointments, meetings I'm going to
attend, and a schedule of routine activities that I'm supposed
to do each day for my recovery.

Sometimes after a flare-up of pain, I remember some essential
detail of my program that I'd completely forgotten about. Rather
than get into a shame-spiral, I simply write down the elements
of my program that I need to practice consistently, and make a
checklist of activities for myself, similar to what a treatment center
or hospital would provide for me. I become my own parent, my
own provider. I take responsibility for my own recovery.

*I'll make sure I have a checklist, if even on a scrap of paper that
I tape to my bathroom mirror—making sure I remember what is
important for me to do each day.*

HONESTY

EMOTIONAL BALANCE

....

"O, Great Spirit, help me always to speak
the truth quietly, to listen with an open mind when
others speak, and to remember the peace
that may be found in silence."

Cherokee prayer

How honest is too honest? I still don't know for sure, and sometimes
I feel like my honesty is just another form of complaining.
Sometimes I can feel that people don't want me to tell them how
I'm feeling all the time or that they're getting tired of hearing about
it. Maybe those closest to me *are* getting tired of hearing about it.
Or maybe it's the way I talk about my pain, or the number of times
I mention it, that wears out those around me.

The nature of my disease is to make me selfish, fearful, resentful,
and dishonest. When I don't get the feedback or support I'm
looking for, my instinct is to isolate, because in isolation I can
nurture my fears and turn them into resentments. This is dishonest,
because if I were to look at myself honestly, I'd realize that the
people around me—family, friends, or caregivers—are doing
their best. It's up to me to be responsible for my recovery. This
means working my program, asking for help when I really
do need help, but doing for myself all the things that I can.
Honesty enables me to do this.

*I practice honesty in my everyday life, and the circle of friends and
family with whom I can be honest without fear is ever-expanding.*

ACTIONS

SPIRITUAL BALANCE

"I have always thought the actions of men
the best interpreters of their thoughts."
John Locke

Spirituality is not something that one has, so much as it is
something that one practices. To be spiritual in my life I need to
remember that it means taking action for my spirit. I can focus
on my body through exercise, and my mind through reading and
journaling, but in order to have balance in my life I need to take
action for my spiritual growth and well-being.

The easiest action I can take to help me in the spiritual part of
my life is praying and meditating on a regular basis. Sometimes
my prayer can be as simple as just talking to my higher power and
asking for strength for today. Sitting still and meditating may be
easier on some days than on others, but on days when I have a lot
of physical pain, I simply make the effort to sit and dedicate a few
moments to meditating—receiving strength from my higher power.

*I am conscious of the actions I am taking for my spiritual well-being
and maintenance. I remember that I am taking action in my life
by making sure that I have prayed and meditated today, regardless
of how I am feeling.*

REACHING OUT

RELATIONSHIPS

....

"A critical element of my pain recovery is developing
relationships within which I can build mutual support
and allies. My twelve-step fellowship provides me
with mutual support and allies to help me stay in pain
recovery. Working the Twelve Steps is an excellent way
to assist me in finding balance. The underlying principles
of the Twelve Steps work for me."
Adapted from Pain Recovery: How to Find Balance
and Reduce Suffering from Chronic Pain

I have many tools today to help me reach out to others in the course
of my pain recovery. Meetings, sponsorship, therapy, and being of
service all take me out of myself and allow me to connect to others,
some of whom I help and some of whom help me. I can give and
receive help today in the spirit of the Twelve Steps. I know that I
can't keep the recovery that I've found unless I give it away to others
who are also in need. This means regular meeting attendance,
fellowshipping with other members, reaching out my hand to
a newcomer, and generally being of service when asked or when
I see a need. My focus is no longer only on myself. I look outward
and see my fellow human beings, and in doing so, I see that
I really do have a place in the world.

*For me to be successful in pain recovery I must be an active and willing
participant in the process. I reach out to others in my twelve-step
program, attend meetings, and work the steps.*

WORKING AND
BEING SELF-SUPPORTING

PHYSICAL BALANCE

....

"When we work hard at the important things
to enrich our lives, our sense of satisfaction is
often hard to describe."
Of Character: Building Assets in Recovery

In recovery, I have found ways to be a productive member
of society. Not only have I found ways to do so, but in the process
of doing so I'm actually helping to maintain balance in many
others areas of my life.

It is easy to get lazy or to fall back on old behavior. Perhaps I'm
out of work—have I done any footwork to get a job? Even if I can't
find a job, there are ways to be self-supporting. Am I contributing
around the house, or am I sitting and watching TV all day and then
complaining about not finding work? Maybe there are tasks around
the house or small projects that have been waiting for someone to
find the time to perform. I can take small steps to help finish such
tasks. I can be productive and get into action regardless of whether
I'm working at a regular job or not. I can communicate regularly
with the people I'm living with to figure out what it would take for
me to be making a contribution to the running of the household.

*I make sure I'm working (even if not at a regular job), being active
and self-supporting. I am contributing to the world that I live in
and I'm not just a taker today.*

CHANGING THE
BRAIN AND PRACTICE

MENTAL BALANCE

....

"Researchers have found that as the brain responds
differently, it physically changes and becomes different.
Emotion and pain have caused the brain to change."
A Day without Pain

Practice makes perfect. Athletes and artists have known this for
thousands of years. A painter sketches a hundred times. The pianist
gets it right on the thousandth note. The athlete throws the ten-
thousandth ball. They may never get it exactly right, but they are
always striving for that perfect stroke, the perfect tone, the perfect
distance. They don't just like the sport, the art, or the music; they
love the practice. They love the process of making that groove in
their mind to help them see the angel in the block of stone, to
hear the series of notes that have not been strung together yet, to
stretch the bounds of the human body. It's the end result of practice
that makes a man stand in wonder and awe. It's witnessing myself
changing my malleable brain, through repetition, into something
more than it was before, something capable of subconsciously
climbing higher, diving deeper, singing louder, and being greater,
that inspires me to continue to work for my recovery.

*The human brain is capable of great things. I am inspired to train
my brain to do that which I had only dreamed of before. Through
repetition, I achieve the excellence I seek.*

MEDITATION

EMOTIONAL BALANCE

....

"Meditation is the soul's perspective glass."
Owen Feltham

Like many things that are good for me, meditation doesn't always feel good. It gets better over time, but in the beginning it's important not to give up. I have found that I can practice meditating regularly for some period of time and then I hit a plateau in my recovery. During those times of struggle I find that practicing meditation may be more difficult, perhaps because I'm feeling things that may be uncomfortable. That in itself is a sign that meditation is having its desired effect. But progressive recovery requires digging deeper, exploring more, and discovering things that were once prevented from coming to the surface by too many other "more pressing" matters. I will be able to deal with these newly uncovered feelings by means of the continued dedication to meditation and prayer.

I continue to meditate, and dedicate some time each day to that important part of my recovery, especially when I least want to do it because of how I'm feeling—I remind myself that consistent meditation will result in long-term improvements to how I feel.

EXERCISE

PHYSICAL BALANCE

....

"Exercise and application produce order in our affairs,
health of body, cheerfulness of mind, and these make
us precious to our friends."
Thomas Jefferson

An essential part of my spiritual connection to my higher self and
higher power is exercise. I understand that exercise and continued
movement are essential to living with chronic pain, free from
the abuse of pain medication and active addiction. Chronic pain
hampered my willingness and ability to exercise. In recovery,
I know better. I strive to exercise in spite of the fear-ridden voice
telling me that I cannot. I don't overdo it when exercising because
that is also unbalanced. I understand I must do some physical
activity on a consistent basis if I'm to continue to maintain a
spiritual connection. I know I have limitations. I respect and
acknowledge them, but I do not use them as a reason for inaction.
I do some form of exercise even if I'm sitting, reclining, or unable
to walk. I learn from physical therapists what I can do that is
within my range of motion and activity. Creativity allows me
to find a way. Consistent movement enables me to grow
and better tolerate my chronic pain.

*I do some form of exercise daily as a way to maintain my spiritual
connection between my higher power and myself. I go easy on myself,
but I make the effort to exercise in some manner. I seek to make
progress and not achieve perfection, taking a step daily to my edge,
but never to pain, closer to my higher power.*

NONJUDGMENTAL

RELATIONSHIPS

·····

*"How seldom we weigh our neighbor
in the same balance as ourselves."*

Thomas à Kempis

I don't like it when others judge me harshly, so I work on resisting the urge to pass judgment on them. Negatively judging others is counterproductive and unhealthy.

Being nonjudgmental means I'm tolerant of opinions and actions of others that don't concern or affect me. It means I disagree with others but respect their right to their own views and perspectives. Being nonjudgmental doesn't mean accepting actions or behaviors from others that threaten my own recovery. I use my discernment to discover those who have the recovery I'd like to emulate. Does this mean I judge or condemn those whose recovery is not quite what I want? Not at all; I just choose not to include them in my close circle. For my recovery to be successful, it's paramount to determine what it means to me. I know that as long as I don't unfairly judge others, I can achieve freedom from feeling judged by others. Acceptance, forgiveness, and humility replace the void that is left when being judgmental departs.

I review my actions and motives. I resist the urge to judge others harshly. Time and energy spent judging others is put to better use in my recovery. My stress diminishes and many things become possible when I'm nonjudgmental and focused on my pain recovery.

DEPRESSION AND GRIEF
EMOTIONAL BALANCE

"The therapist counseled me about compound grief and how difficult it was to deal with. I cried constantly and as I did I could hear my disease voice telling me to be embarrassed and to shut down the feelings. Somehow I knew if I didn't feel everything I needed to feel, I wouldn't survive. If I attempted in any way to shut down those feelings, I would end up either relapsing or killing myself."
Tails of Recovery: Addicts and the Pets That Love Them

The short-term suppression of a sad feeling may be necessary for me to get through a task and do what needs to be done, but the suppression of multiple deeper feelings, especially over a period of time, is depression or repression of feelings. In recovery, freedom comes from feeling my feelings, realizing they cannot hurt me, working through them, then getting to the other side, stronger than before.

Today I know that I don't need to lash out when I feel the flicker of depression, and I also know that there is an antidote to this deadly emotional state, and it's summed up in one word: action. My physical balance works together with my emotional balance to help me take necessary action to lift my depression. Just knowing that there is something I can do about the feeling of depression helps take away some of its power to hurt me.

OPEN-MINDEDNESS

MENTAL BALANCE

....

"As our understanding of pain grows, researchers now describe pain as not just a mind-body phenomenon, but one in which psychological, social, and spiritual factors, as well as biological ones, must be taken into consideration."
A Day without Pain

My pain affected all areas of my life. So must my recovery. I trust this is not just philosophy or lofty thinking. This is practical, research-supported, professionally accepted thinking. Twelve-step recovery has worked for many people. It can work for me. All I need is to stay open-minded to the knowledge that there are a great many people out there who do care. They have dedicated years of their own lives studying what it is that I suffer from. It's hard to believe sometimes, because in active addiction I felt so alone. It seemed like no one understood. I know today that others have been down the same road as me. They have found recovery. They continue to help others find recovery. All I need is to get out of my own way and let my spirit connect with that of others in recovery. I see what they do, I listen to their words, and strive to remain open-minded and let the healing process happen.

I must keep my mind open to the spirit that exists, a spirit that is the solution to problems my mind and body alone cannot help.

PATIENCE

EMOTIONAL BALANCE

"The first step in this program is to recognize that your pain is no longer just physical, but also emotional and spiritual. You need to reconnect with your emotions, your body, and your spirit. You benefit by allowing yourself to be open to the possibility of real, lasting relief without medication. Living with pain in this way is a process, and it takes time."

A Day without Pain

Finding emotional balance and harmony requires patience. Often it feels like everything I do for my program is what I do "in the meantime." The balance I'm seeking does not come simply because I want it, and it does not always come quickly. It is not something I get of my own free will and desire. If that were true, I would be able to just "will away" my chronic pain and "will in" balance and harmony within myself. Instead, it requires work over time—in other words, patience. This I am willing to have and to practice today.

I'm seeking balance and harmony in my emotions, and during that journey I accept that I may feel pain during this process. I also accept that the recovery of my wounded spirit may take time, but I will recover.

EMOTIONS AND THE SPIRIT

SPIRITUAL BALANCE

....

"Let's not forget that the little emotions are the great captains of our lives and we obey them without realizing it."
Vincent Van Gogh

I've heard it said many times that the longest journey is the one within, or from the head to the heart. I can work on all of the things outside myself that I want or think I need, but the journey within, the strength I find inside, and the connection with that spirit within me have the greatest and most direct impact on all other points of balance, emotional, mental, and physical. When I take the time to focus on my meditation, prayer, and being of service, I find I am able to handle my emotions and keep them within an acceptable range.

Sometimes events may trigger my emotions to spike, but those emotions do not need to stay at an unpleasant, elevated level for nearly as long as they used to. When I remember to stay spiritually focused and pray for help, my emotions do not have the destructive power to run my life they once had. I recall that sometimes I even made important decisions when in a highly emotional state. I don't do that today.

Today I seek out my higher power in prayer first, I allow my emotions to settle, and then I make decisions later, from a more guided and centered place.

When my emotions begin to "spike," I focus on my spiritual connection, allowing my emotions to settle into a reasonable, manageable range, and only when I am calm and centered do I return to the issue I was dealing with when my emotions spiked in the first place.

PHYSICAL INTIMACY

RELATIONSHIPS

*"Sexual activity is a normal part of intimacy
and need not be given up."*
Pain Recovery: How to Find Balance and
Reduce Suffering from Chronic Pain

Reigniting intimacy can actually help reduce my pain and suffering. During orgasm, the body floods with endorphins, and this can help relieve my pain. Trying different positions or activities other than traditional intercourse may be satisfying and enhance intimacy without causing pain. I can think creatively with my sexual partner about how to enhance our sex life. (If I don't have a partner, then I can think creatively about how to find one.)

It is completely acceptable for me to express my concerns with my partner. I can share my fears, desires, and limitations. I can tell my partner what is pleasurable and what is not. I know that communication is the key. This communication is often best accomplished outside the bedroom.

I'm conscious of the fact that having a healthy sex life can be just as important a part of my recovery as other areas of my life. Healthy sexuality helps maintain the four points of balance. I look at achieving that healthy sex life as another component of my pain recovery.

24

APPRECIATING
WHAT I CAN DO

PHYSICAL BALANCE

....

"Next to excellence is the appreciation of it."
William Makepeace Thackeray

It's true; I cannot do all the things I used to be able to do with ease.
Some days my pain makes it difficult to do much of anything—but
I appreciate the things that I am able to do all the more.

In addition to monitoring my level of pain in order to adjust
my activities appropriately, I make sure I pay attention to the things
I can do today—too much attention to the pain that I have on any
given day can lead me to focus only on the negative. I need balance
in every area of my life today, and remembering to appreciate
the good is a necessary counterweight to monitoring what
is not so good.

I may not be able to dance today, but I can appreciate and
applaud those who can.

*I think of all the things my body can do today, and I regard myself
with appreciation for my abilities, not my disabilities. I have gratitude
in my life today.*

VICIOUS CYCLE

MENTAL BALANCE

....

"The urge but the inability to do something,
anything, to quiet the beast or kill the pain can
become overwhelming. Preoccupation with pain
can lead to a vicious cycle in which the person
enters a state of profound suffering."
A Day without Pain

Suffering can happen whether I'm using and abusing medication
or not. The cycle starts once I start to get out of balance on any one
of the four levels, be it emotional, mental, spiritual, or physical.
The cycle is subtle and can begin with just neglecting (I may call
it forgetting or not having time) to do the things I need to do for
myself to stay in the cycle of recovery. The downward vicious cycle
of being a victim of chronic pain can happen without my noticing
consciously; however, I can also change that cycle at any given
moment of any given day, regardless of what is happening.
At any moment I can shift the cycle and choose to be in pain
recovery rather than being a victim of pain. Awareness and
acknowledgment of the cycles are the first step. I stay aware
of this tendency to follow the cycle of victim-thinking so
that it doesn't become self-perpetuating.

*I regularly ask myself what cycle I'm in: the vicious, downward
cycle of addiction and victim-thinking or the upward, recovery
cycle of pain recovery.*

NOURISHING MYSELF

PHYSICAL BALANCE

"What we eat every day has a profound effect on how
we feel. Our foods play a major role in our health and
well-being. Scientists and researchers have concluded
that a poor diet contributes to a third of all cancers."

A Day without Pain

It's no secret that the foods we eat can affect the way we feel.
Too much or too little of certain nutrients and substances can throw
me out of physical balance. Even a simple digestive upset can make
my chronic pain worse. And eating certain "comfort" foods might
really just be a way of stuffing my feelings, so I need to be aware
of occasions when I might be doing "emotional eating" rather
than eating for nutrition.

If something I eat doesn't feel right or make me feel good, then I
stop eating it. One too many fast-food burgers, large fries, and large
"diet" sodas; one too many instances when I feel like I can't move
after I eat—these are signs that I'm not paying attention to my body.
I take care of me today by listening to the advice of nutritionists,
doctors, and others who have studied the effects of foods that help
fight pain. Today I choose foods that give me energy and strength.

*How I feel is more important than the instant gratification of
what tastes good. I'm caring for myself by taking care in what
I put into my body today.*

FORGIVENESS

SPIRITUAL BALANCE

··

"No child of God sins to that degree as to
make himself incapable of forgiveness."
John Bunyan

I work to discover the true meaning of self-forgiveness. The
emotional pain, which accompanies my physical chronic pain,
hinders and distorts my ability to view myself in a positive light.
By working a pain recovery program, working the Twelve Steps,
attending meetings, talking with others in recovery, reading, and
writing, I work to forgive myself on a daily basis for that which
I *cannot* control, *cannot* change, and *cannot* yet accept. The
emotional pain of self-blame and self-loathing drains my life's
energy, energy that could be better used for healing. I work on my
recovery so that I don't have to regret my past and forgive myself
for past wrongs and mistakes. I make amends as the steps direct me
to do, and when I make or live my amends, my guilt and shame
subside and self-forgiveness is possible. I'm no longer stuck in the
downward spiral of darkness, despair, shame, and guilt; instead I'm
in a cycle of recovery, working daily to achieve forgiveness, finding
love and light within myself and others.

*Through the tools I've gained in recovery I'm practicing self-forgiveness
on a daily basis. I feel good about myself and learn to cut myself some
slack. I'm all I have, for without me I cannot hope to do the good work
I know I want to do to help myself and others to grow in recovery.*

HABITS

RELATIONSHIPS

....

"Happiness is a habit—cultivate it."
Elbert Hubbard

Today I practice the habits of recovery in my life, which include
working hard, arriving where I've said I'd be on time, participating
in family activities, and refraining from gossip, to name just a few.
I'm also making a habit of maintaining relationships in my life
and sharing with others what I've learned. Sharing with others helps
me maintain my own recovery. I make sure to share happy news
as well as sad, and I rejoice with others in their happiness. That
is part of sharing, too.

*I share the habits that work for me with those in my recovery support
group and I let them see how I go about improving the areas I want
to improve. Sharing with others not only helps them, but it also
strengthens my own recovery.*

TOLERANCE

PHYSICAL BALANCE

"Good humor makes all things possible."
Henry Ward Beecher

When my physical therapist or other medical professional urges me to push myself just a little harder than I want to, I remember that he or she is helping to develop my tolerance for activity and I cooperate to the best of my ability instead of reacting by whining or pleading that I can't do it.

My pain may limit me physically at times, and some days may be worse than others, but the longer I live with the pain, the more I'm able to tolerate it. The more I can tolerate, the less debilitated I am by my pain. I learn to accept the good with the bad and also acknowledge the strength that living with chronic pain has given me. No matter what the circumstances on any given day, I devote myself to the solution. I owe it to myself to be proactive in my own pain recovery.

I learn to tolerate my pain in increments, pushing my limits a little further each day. This is the way I grow and regain function to the best of my ability.

IMBALANCE OF THOUGHTS

MENTAL BALANCE

....

"When I have pain it often sets off unbalanced thinking.
When I'm hurting, my thinking becomes distorted.
During these times I'm tempted to think of using opioids
to relieve my pain. During times when my pain flares,
I may think that I've had enough pain and that using
drugs is the only thing that will help, even though my
experience is that using drugs has in some ways only
increased my pain over a period of time and severely
affected my quality of life. In pain it's easy to forget
where I came from because of the confusion the pain
creates. I can forget how I ended up being controlled
by the medication that was supposed to treat the
pain that was controlling me and my life. When
I'm in enough pain I may even tell myself that it
will be different this time."

Adapted from Pain Recovery: How to Find Balance
and Reduce Suffering from Chronic Pain

It is not a matter of whether I may have these thoughts, but when,
because it is natural for them to come up. But during these times
when I'm looking for the easy solution or quick fix, I see that there
are other, better options for me that work over time.

*I remember that pain itself can affect my thinking. The actions I take
today are the actions I put in place before the pain gets so bad that it
affects my thinking. Once my thinking is affected, I trust the action
plan I put in place before this happened.*

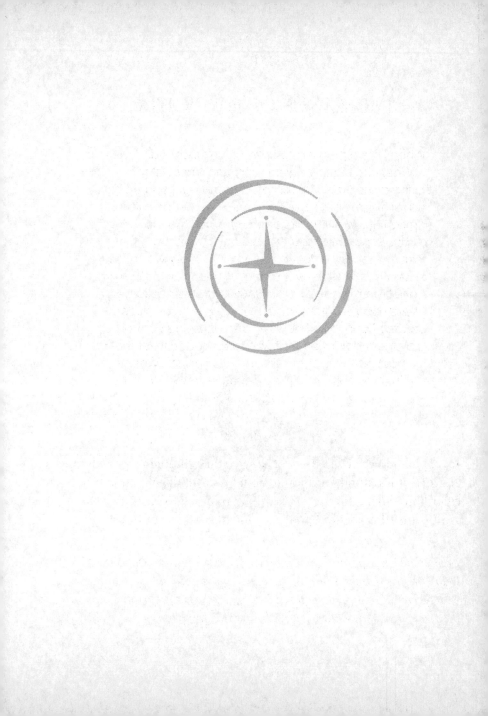

{ DECEMBER }

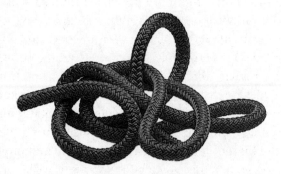

SERENITY

EMOTIONAL BALANCE

....

*"Becoming aware of what you are feeling
and trying to honestly and calmly assess what is
happening can help you deal with your pain."*
A Day without Pain

The instant something happened to me in the past, whether it was good or bad, I would completely spike in my emotional reaction to it. Healthy emotions range between a four and a seven on a ten-point scale. If I'm in one, two, or three, I'm in depression. If I'm in eight, nine, or ten, I'm overly elated. It takes some time for my emotions to calm back down.

In active addiction, I thought I had to act right away in order to get the emotions under control, suppress them, keep them inside. Surrender means allowing the emotions to come and go. It means that I allow myself the time to calm down. I let my emotions come back into a manageable range and then take action from there. During the time when I'm vulnerable to a flare-up of pain, I'm also vulnerable to acting on addiction, making mistakes, causing damage, hurting myself and others. During these times I use the tools of recovery first. I pray to my higher power, meditate, go to a meeting, call my sponsor, write, or read. From that place, I take action.

Everything can wait except recovery. No decision is so important that it must be made right away when I'm in a heightened emotional state.

FLEXIBILITY

SPIRITUAL BALANCE

"Everything is changeable, everything appears and disappears; there is no blissful peace until one passes beyond the agony of life and death."

Siddhartha Gautama, the Buddha

Everything changes: A signpost of spiritual balance in my life is the ability to be flexible regarding situations in my life. Even my physical flexibility is largely dependent on my spiritual condition. Am I breathing deeply? Am I remembering that recovery is about progress and not perfection? Am I allowing my spiritual connection to my higher power to evolve and develop over time? Am I holding too rigidly to some idea or concept that is not working for me?

Recovery changes me. These changes make it possible for me to live without the use of drugs. Today it's possible for me to accept my pain, to embrace it as part of myself and not resist it; but that change has only been possible as a result of tapping into something more powerful than myself. I maintain my contact with that power, so that when I have days when my pain flares up, my spiritual condition is intact, strong, and ready and able to support me through that process. I invite my spirit into my mental, emotional, and physical work, always remembering that the entire process is made much easier when I'm spiritually centered, connected, and flexible.

I look at the way my spiritual connection fluctuates, remembering that I have the ability to be flexible, to change and allow that connection to grow. I look at the areas of my spiritual practice that are too rigid as well as those areas that could use more rigidity.

RECEIVING

RELATIONSHIPS

....

"I must surrender in order to win. I live 'just for today'
so I may enjoy tomorrow. I admit powerlessness to
become empowered. I give so I may receive."
Tails of Recovery: Addicts and the Pets That Love Them

In the book *Pain Recovery*, I looked at giving and receiving. I have
grown in this area and can look at the way some of the things that
stood in my way at one point are now different, while there are still
other areas that I must work on. How do I feel about others helping
me today? In recovery it can become more difficult to ask for help
because I may feel like I should be further along or I am afraid of
what others will think of me if I do ask.

What are my barriers to receiving help from others today? What
can I do to overcome these issues?

*I take a look at my challenges in receiving, as well as the qualities that
make it easier to receive, help from others—how far I have come and
how much further I have to go in being able to accept their help.*

STRENGTH

PHYSICAL BALANCE

"That which does not kill me, makes me stronger."
Friedrich Nietzsche

If I choose to allow my pain to take precedence in my life, I can become filled with self-pity. I give strength to my chronic pain and weaken my pain recovery when I start asking questions like "Why me? What did I do to deserve this?" Even in recovery I can find myself sinking into despair and allowing my responsibilities to fall by the wayside. However, life goes on. There are chores that have to be handled, bills that need to be paid, and perhaps other people who count on me to be there for them. Instead of wallowing in misery I summon the personal strength I find through maintaining physical balance and am able to focus on what I am capable of doing and do it to the best of my ability. If I need to take several breaks during the day to gain back my strength, then that is okay, because I know at the end of the day I have not wasted my time doing nothing and feeling sorry for myself. I focus on my strengths and what I am capable of accomplishing instead of allowing self-pity to immobilize me.

I draw strength from within by focusing on maintaining physical balance. From that strength I find the ability to move forward through the trying times in life, and have the ability to live another day in recovery, regardless of how my pain is behaving.

SPIRITUALITY

MENTAL BALANCE

··

"Spirituality pertains to the intellectual or
higher endowments of the mind or soul."
A Day without Pain

As I progress in my recovery, my definition of spirituality changes
with each spiritual awakening I experience. Awareness increases.
Contact and connection strengthen. Each awakening offers a
deeper understanding. Spirituality is the intention to find inner
connection to a power greater than myself. It is the desire and the
ability to move from one place to another within me. In my search,
quest, and seeking for that power within, I move from one way of
being, acting, or doing to another. I try different things. I work on
different aspects of my spirituality. I pray differently, meditate using
different techniques, always working to find things that work for me.

*My spirituality is open to my own interpretation, but it is what
I'm doing between each spiritual awakening, what I do with what
is offered to me during the spiritual awakening.*

EXPECTATIONS

EMOTIONAL BALANCE

....

"Patients who are given inactive substances
and told these substances would take away
the pain respond to the placebo."
A Day without Pain

I can get so stuck in my emotions that they in some way become
another form of drug for me. I get addicted to drama, as I once did
to the secondary gain of my active addiction. I can become addicted
to the attention my pain gets me, to anything that distracts me from
reality—a reality I must face instead of escaping. I face reality by
working steps. When I'm stuck in these negative feelings, I need
to believe and expect the emotional pain will go away. Feelings
change. The reason a placebo works is because patients *expect* that
it will work, they hope it will work, they have desire that it will
work. I have desire, hope, and an expectation that what I'm doing
for my pain recovery helps with my emotions. That gives me a
much better chance to experience that it does work. Recovery is
working for me today—it is literally changing the way I feel.
Just knowing that I'm doing something, whether or not the actual
act in and of itself is enough to heal or "fix" me, I expect that
it will, and sometimes that is enough.

*I expect recovery to help me feel joy, peace, serenity; I expect the
things I do to change the way I feel.*

BEING AWARE OF THE POSITIVE

SPIRITUAL BALANCE

....

"As we've discussed, the sheer discomfort of chronic pain often results in negative thought patterns. One form these thoughts can take is to ignore, dismiss, or otherwise not be aware of anything remotely positive about this situation, whatever it may be. With or without my knowledge, I end up focusing all my conscious attention and energy on the negative aspects of the situation. For example, I hear from ten people how well I seem to be doing, while a single person tells me, for whatever reason, I don't seem to be doing well. Rather than believe the ten people with positive views, I'm certain the one negative perspective is correct. In addition to feeding my negativity, this can also serve the self-defeating purpose of confirming what I believe about myself—that I'm not doing well. I find evidence in real events to support the position I've already taken."

Adapted from Pain Recovery: How to Find Balance
and Reduce Suffering from Chronic Pain

I keep in mind that nearly all situations and events have both positive and negative characteristics. Sometimes I may have to look a little harder or even do some work to locate the positive, but if I search for it, I find it. Something else I can do to counteract negative thinking is to identify things or people I'm grateful for. Practicing and expressing gratitude can improve mood and measurably increase the experience of happiness.

I identify things or people I'm grateful for and make sure I know the reasons for my gratitude.

RECOVERY

RELATIONSHIPS

....

"As we learn to be responsible for our recovery while
accepting help from others, we develop the ability
to have peers. We learn that in the same relationship,
often within the course of minutes or hours, we can
both accept and offer help."

Of Character: Building Assets in Recovery

Recovery is a process. Friends, family, and others who are
supportive of my recovery are helpful, but finding others who have
experience with the new path I'm on provides the type of support
I need rather than just sympathy for my "plight." Building mutual
support and alliances, I avail myself of the personal and spiritual
growth that comes from others sharing their experience, strength,
and hope with me. I give myself permission to receive help from
others. Being able to receive requires admitting there are some
things I can't and shouldn't attempt to do on my own. And I know
that I won't always be on the receiving end, but that I will gladly
help others when it's my turn to do so.

*I ask for and accept assistance from those who have experience in
areas in which I need help. I look to my twelve-step program and pain
recovery support group as I build relationships with those who have
come before me, as well as those who follow me.*

SPIRITUAL AWAKENING

PHYSICAL BALANCE

....

"No human being ever learns to live until he has
awakened to the dormant powers within him."
William James

A spiritual awakening can consist of remembering to maintain
physical balance even during the darkest or most painful of
moments. Through this awakening and focus on my physical
balance, even when in severe pain, I have gotten through the day,
will continue to get through life, and do not need to abuse pain
medication. Regardless of the type of pain I'm feeling, the spiritual
awakening I have discovered in recovery is enabling me to keep
the focus on my physical well-being.

In desperate times my thoughts lead back to the old idea of taking
pain medication to "take the edge off." I have to think through the
entire process of what will happen if I return to abusing medication
or using other drugs. All my past experiences show that every time
I abused pain medication, it always led to more—an insatiable
need. My faith and trust in a higher power carries me through those
moments today. The spiritual power within carries me through.
I am awake to that power today.

*I appreciate the spiritual awakenings I have received and continue
to receive in pain recovery, not the least of which is knowing that
regardless of the type of pain I'm feeling on any given day, I focus
first on my physical balance, health, and well-being.*

ATTITUDE
MENTAL BALANCE

....

*"There is nothing either good or bad,
but thinking makes it so."*
William Shakespeare

Thinking rigidly, in either/or terms, where things are either one
extreme or another with nothing in between, creates imbalance
in my life. When I'm like this I view events, situations, and people
in one of only two mutually exclusive ways: all good or all bad.
Everything is either great or it's horrible.

When my attitude is black-and-white it means that I think in
extremes—either I am perfect or I am a total failure. I am in
constant pain or I must be totally pain-free. My attitude can shift
from one extreme to the other, depending on circumstances. In
this thought pattern there is no middle ground. In fact, most reality
occurs somewhere in the middle, neither black nor white but
within shades of gray. When I'm unable to appreciate the gray area,
I end up missing much of the richness of life. I regain balance in
recovery by becoming consciously aware of this tendency, checking
my attitude and noticing when I'm thinking in black-and-white
terms. This awareness continues to provide me with the opportunity
to look for the middle ground. Today, I'm not in pain all the time,
and I'm not completely comfortable all the time. I'm in the
gray area, and that's okay.

*I pay attention to my black-and-white thinking, remembering that
recovery is sometimes in the shades of gray.*

FAITH

EMOTIONAL BALANCE

*"Research has proven that when someone
is afraid, their pain scores increase. Conversely,
teaching people to reduce their fear about
a situation can decrease their pain."*
A Day without Pain

The reality is that I can't act in fear and act in faith at the same time. I'm acting in fear when I stay home, stay in bed, don't go for a walk, to work, or to a meeting because I'm afraid of the pain that I *may* experience when I do. I'm acting in faith when I ask my higher power for help and, to the best of my ability, I go about performing the functions and duties that I had scheduled. I may not be able to perform them to the fullest extent possible, but I do what I can, having faith—and that shifts my emotions. It shifts my feelings about the situation and diminishes the pain that I can feel when I give up or give in to my fear.

*I know I can act out of fear or act in faith. I choose to act
in faith, knowing when I do that pretty soon my emotions
will match the actions.*

GRATITUDE

SPIRITUAL BALANCE

"Another important part of the maintenance of pain recovery is cultivating an attitude of gratitude for whatever blessings I have. Sometimes I may have to look a little harder to see the blessings in my life, but there are always things to be grateful for, no matter how desperate the situation seems. I can learn, perhaps to my surprise, that it is possible to remain in conscious contact with gratitude in spite of feelings of physical pain, anger, depression, or fear."

Adapted from Pain Recovery: How to Find Balance
and Reduce Suffering from Chronic Pain

The balancing effects of enhanced spirituality and its positive impact on my pain recovery may become apparent only gradually over time. It can be weeks or even months after these processes first begin before I realize that my awareness, feelings, and behavior have started to change. When I build a balanced foundation of spirituality that is based on hope, trust, and faith, I maximize both my internal harmony and the potential for harmony between myself and others.

By focusing on gratitude during the process of growth and change, I allow the principles of hope, trust, and faith to take hold and give me comfort during the sometimes challenging and painful process of growing.

GIVING

RELATIONSHIPS

···

"Give a little love to a child,
and you get a great deal back."
John Ruskin

Am I ready to give back to others? This can start the very first day I'm in recovery. Whatever my particular circumstance, giving starts on day one and does not end. Giving completes the circle of balanced relationships. But I must *have* something in order to give it away. Many people think of giving back in terms of time, money, and resources. This is part of giving, but so is giving back my experience of how I achieved recovery and balance in my life. Rather than giving advice, I share solutions and my experience, strength, and hope. I freely give to others what I have received, out of appreciation for what others have given me.

The ability to give back is a gift that recovery provides. When I "get out of myself" it helps me to see my problems in the proper perspective and context. It allows me to focus on things in my life for which I can be grateful. And the most wonderful thing about giving is that although I have learned to give without thought of return, I gain a great deal more than I give to others when I share my experience, strength, and hope with them.

I give to another person what I have been given—not the time, money,
or resources so much as the shared experience of freedom from addictive
medications to manage my pain.

IMBALANCE OF PHYSICAL LIFE

PHYSICAL BALANCE

"Imbalance of the body can manifest as fatigue, aching, sleep disturbance, and increased pain."
Pain Recovery: How to Find Balance and
Reduce Suffering from Chronic Pain

Stopping opioids caused an upheaval for a period of time, and balance was difficult to achieve until my body recovered its own store of endorphins. This may be an ongoing process that takes some time, even now. It's important for me to work on balance during this time to offset the physical discomfort that is part of withdrawal. This can also happen when I make changes in my life in pain recovery, such as increased activity or returning to work. During these times and changes it is critical to get support in other parts of my recovery—thoughts, emotions, and spirituality.

Maintaining balance in my physical life means continuing to monitor but not judge my state of nutrition, energy, exercise patterns, and toxins. I need to avoid extremes. If I exercise too much I can burn out. If my diet is too rigid I eventually eat unhealthy foods. Balance means monitoring my body as well as my emotions.

I review my action plan for physical imbalance; when I'm tired, when I'm in more pain, when I can't sleep, or when I have other physical problems, I have a series of actions in place in advance and am committed to taking them.

SPIRITUALITY

MENTAL BALANCE

"One hour's meditation on the work of the Creator
is better than seventy years of prayer."
The Quran

When was the last time I meditated? Maybe it was only
yesterday or maybe it has been days, weeks, or months. However
long it has been, I can always recommit myself to the process.
I can even meditate more than once a day if I like, with a
renewed focus and commitment.

During my meditation I think about what I am doing: I am taking
time out of my day and dedicating it to my spiritual path, to my
recovery, to my body, mind, and soul. As I breathe in and out,
thinking about my higher power, I feel my own restlessness, anxiety,
or pain, and breathe through it. Through this practice I strengthen
my own ability to sit through my feelings and sit with my pain. I
take five, ten, or twenty minutes to sit with my pain and make it
my friend. I do not add to my own suffering by hating, resisting, or
abusing that part of myself that is in pain.

*Through my practice I sit with my feelings and strengthen
my connection to myself and to my higher power.*

TOLERANCE

EMOTIONAL BALANCE

....

"It is the emotional experience of pain that has been
shown to be especially important to our perception of
pain and, ultimately, our suffering."
A Day without Pain

The difference between pain and suffering is perception.
The emotional pain I feel as a result of my chronic pain comes
from my resistance to the chronic pain. It's normal and natural
to grieve the loss of function. This grief can take years to work
through. But the way I experience my chronic pain is what affects
my emotional pain. Self-pity and feeling like a victim just make the
pain worse. The feelings that friends and family shy away from are
not the physical, chronic pain feelings. It's the emotional anguish
that follows. No one wants to be around someone who has a cork
in the bottle of emotions, as they are easily transferred to others.
People can feel those suppressed feelings when they walk into
the room I'm in. I don't ask others to feel my feelings for me today.
I take responsibility for my condition. I express my feelings;
I accept my chronic pain; I move forward into acceptance,
forgiveness, and recovery.

*Acceptance and forgiveness of my chronic pain, expression of
my emotional pain, is freedom. I practice acceptance, forgiveness,
and expression so that I can get a proper perspective on and
tolerance for my chronic pain.*

NONJUDGMENTAL

SPIRITUAL BALANCE

....

"When we are accepting in recovery, we 'receive' others, the world, our circumstances, and ourselves 'as adequate.' This does not mean we must be content with things exactly as they are. It means we learn to align ourselves with and acknowledge reality. Only when we have done so are we able to develop the wisdom to know when we can work to change things and when we must learn to accept things as they are."

Of Character: Building Assets in Recovery

Expectations usually involve judging myself, others, and situations against specific standards for behavior and a reality that I've constructed in my mind. Sometimes these expectations become imperatives, such as "things must be the way I want them to be." Whenever I think in terms of how people or situations *should* be and judge the situation or people according to preset standards and beliefs, I'm setting myself up for resentment and disappointment. Do I make an effort not to judge others today?

When I'm feeling like judging situations and other people, I look at my own expectations, behaviors, and standards I'm setting. I discover what I'm trying to get out of a situation and a loving way to provide that for myself.

WHOLENESS

RELATIONSHIPS

"Love is as simple, yet demanding, as seeing the
parts of our loved ones' personalities that are not
as we would like them to be and accepting and loving
them as whole people without having to make excuses
or redecorate the reality of who they are....
Love is based on connection at its most whole
and most spiritual level."

Of Character: Building Assets in Recovery

It's challenging for me to accept someone else as a whole person when I don't feel whole myself. Part of me was lost to active addiction, another part to chronic pain. But today, through pain recovery, I am recovering those parts of me that were lost; I've been able to work toward reclaiming, or recovering, those parts of me that were lost to abusing medication and the behavior that followed. As I reclaim and recover those parts of me, I look to others and am able to see the wholeness within them. Through shared experiences, exchange of time and energy, and mutual acceptance of self and the other, intimacy is created. I no longer feel the need to complete myself with other people. My program of recovery completes me, so I'm free to love another without needing them to complete me.

I am a whole person, recovering those parts of me lost to active addiction. In my wholeness, I see, accept, and love others in my life for the whole person they are. Intimacy is created; spiritual balance is enhanced through my intimacy with myself and others.

IMBALANCE OF EMOTIONS, POSITIVE ACTION

EMOTIONAL BALANCE

"When I have challenging situations, particularly around my chronic pain and functioning in the world without drugs, its not uncommon to have negative emotions. Part of using pain medication to treat the pain was also using it to treat the emotions that came with the pain. Without using medication when I experience emotional imbalance it comes in the form of fear, anger, anxiety, sadness, and frustration; but I also find that I can feel more excitement, happiness, and elation. I'm not used to dealing with these feelings.... Unless I know what I'm feeling I can become a victim to the feelings and have no power to handle them."

A Day without Pain

The antidote to negative emotions is action; but negative emotions can make it difficult for me to even *think* of taking action. I can become trapped in a vicious cycle of negative feelings if I allow this to happen. But the tools of pain recovery, if I remember to use them, can break the cycle. I "get out of myself": I call a sponsor, a counselor, a friend in recovery; do something for someone else; read recovery literature; attend a meeting; work steps. I don't allow my negative emotions to carry me down into a repetitive cycle of pain.

It takes hard work for me to change my patterns, and the kind of work I've done so far requires continuous vigilance to sustain the changes I've made. The best way for me to do this is to make sure I've got my action plan in place for when my emotions spike: What positive actions can I take when I get emotionally imbalanced?

OPEN-MINDEDNESS

MENTAL BALANCE

....

"There are no drawbacks to
seeking a spiritual experience."
Pain Recovery: How to Find Balance and
Reduce Suffering from Chronic Pain

If what I hear from others in my recovery fellowship sounds
strange or odd, in such cases I use my mental faculties to discern
what I can use—and later I may ask a sponsor or trusted friend
in my fellowship to help me understand what sounded odd to me.
There is no harm in listening to the experiences of others. I can
learn from anyone. I understand that while some people may
share their spiritual beliefs with me, I can also share my beliefs
and practices with them. There is no harm in being able to learn
more, hear more, share more, and in so doing get more information
about practices that may work for me—if not now, then
perhaps in the future.

*I seek out more information, knowing it only helps and cannot hurt my
recovery. I listen and learn from what others do in their pain recovery
program. If it seems useful to me, I may incorporate it into my own
beliefs. If not, I let it go. Either way, it cannot hurt me.*

ATTITUDE
EMOTIONAL BALANCE

....

"Mood is inextricably linked to the experience of pain.
Depression is one of the most common components
of Chronic Pain Syndrome (CPS). Chronic pain
and depression are irrevocably linked. CPS causes
depression, depression increases pain."
A Day without Pain

Am I depressed because I'm in pain or am I in pain because I'm depressed? Did I stop meditating and praying before or after my pain became chronic? Did I stop calling my sponsor because I was feeling depressed, or did I get depressed and then stop calling my sponsor? These are questions that may never get answered in recovery, but it's important to ask, to be aware.

I'm no longer anesthetized with drugs; I can actually feel my pain and my moods more acutely now, and I know I must stay the course. As I learn to tolerate my moods better, accept them, address them, identify them, and then move through them in recovery, my pain is lessened. My moods change. I find myself feeling less pain, feeling more joy, and experiencing moods worth sharing and holding onto.

In recovery, I am not afraid of my moods. I work my program regardless of the mood I'm in. The tools of recovery help me work through the way I'm feeling so that I can live a life worth living with my chronic pain.

PERFECTIONISM

SPIRITUAL BALANCE

....

"Perfection falls not to the share of mortals."
George Washington

Whatever perfection is, I know today that perfection is not "purity." For example, I may need to take medication for a medical procedure, or my illness may require it. However, taking that needed medication does not mean that I'm "impure," or not working a perfect program. I work a "good-enough" program, which means I put one foot in front of the other and do the next right thing. Some days are better than others, but the real goal is developing inner strength, an inner relationship, and dialogue with a higher power that gets me through anything life has to offer. I don't get hung up on ideas of purity or definitions of perfection. I know the difference between taking the needed treatment for my illness and taking advantage to feed my disease of addiction. I don't abuse medication today. I don't act out on defects and other addictions. This is perfection for me today. This, today, is spiritual. This, today, is recovery.

I am a perfect child of my higher power, my higher self, in all of my pain, in all of my recovery. When I find the struggle in my physical world, in the mundane and everyday activities of life, to be too much, in those moments I find the perfection within and embrace the idea that perfection outside, externally, is a myth.

AWARENESS

RELATIONSHIPS

....

"Kindness is another character trait often thought of as
old-fashioned or as a soft virtue. Being kind requires we
bring other character traits to bear. In order to be kind,
we must have the ability to notice, consider, and act
on what would be helpful and welcomed by another.
We must be self- and other-aware, and we must be
capable of selflessness and generosity."
Of Character: Building Assets in Recovery

My level of kindness to others has a direct effect on my physical
health. The energy I put out into the world is the energy I get back.
My body needs positive, healing energy, based in love and light,
in order to operate at maximum capacity. I'm already up against a
curve living with chronic pain, and just like I need to be careful
of what I'm putting into my body, watching the way I eat, sleep,
exercise, and participate in my recovery, I also need to be careful
of the energy that is coming into it. I must pay attention to what
I put out, so that I can get that same type of energy back. I want,
need, and desire only the highest and best vibrations, and
nothing can be as healing as kindness.

*I show kindness to others, complete strangers and the closest of
companions, knowing the kindness I show others is the energy I'm
sending to myself. My physical health depends on receiving the energy
of kindness. I receive that energy as it cycles through others, into the
world, through my higher power, and is returned unto me.*

SPIRITUAL IMBALANCE, POSITIVE ACTION

SPIRITUAL BALANCE

"The balancing effects of enhanced spirituality may become apparent only gradually over time. It can be weeks or even months after these processes first begin before you realize that your awareness, feelings, and behavior have started to change. When you build a balanced foundation of spirituality that is based on the cornerstones of hope, trust, and faith, you maximize you're your internal harmony and the potential for harmony between yourself and others."

Pain Recovery for Families: How to Find Balance When Someone Else's Chronic Pain Becomes Your Problem Too

I may swing from one extreme to another from day to day, depending on events, but one thing is steady: my commitment to my recovery. I stay focused on my spiritual practices, such as prayer and meditation, to help me keep all areas of my life and my recovery on track and in balance.

I review and update my spiritual action plan, which is a plan for those times when I feel spiritually unbalanced. I know what I need to do for my recovery during times of crisis.

OPTIMISM

MENTAL BALANCE

....

"Pain is never permanent."

St. Teresa of Avila

I have to be optimistic as I go through my daily life, but not so optimistic that I allow myself to indulge in unrealistic fantasies instead of dealing with reality. One of those fantasies is that my chronic pain will be cured. I can waste my entire life sitting around in bed, overly medicated, waiting for my pain to be cured. But by definition, there is no cure to chronic pain. I can't afford to entertain those fantasies anymore. Acceptance of reality gives me the freedom to move on to the solution. I'm open to new possibilities once I close the door on old ideas. The sooner I accept this, the sooner I can look for solutions. I may have to surrender on a daily basis. I seek out a new way to relieve my pain—one that I have never tried before. I remember to be optimistic, but to leave the results up to my higher power.

Every day I may wake up and think of old ideas, thoughts, or notions, but every day I recommit to closing the door on those old ways of thinking and opening the door that leads to new ways of thought and of living. There are many solutions for people like me who are living with chronic pain and in recovery, which means that today I have options and the willingness to use them.

PATIENCE

SPIRITUAL BALANCE

*"Maintaining the spirituality needed for pain
recovery can require ongoing practice in developing
my understanding of and ability to apply such
principles as patience, tolerance, acceptance,
and humility. Patience is waiting without worrying
and enduring without complaint."*
Adapted from Pain Recovery: How to Find Balance
and Reduce Suffering from Chronic Pain

I do my best, no matter what the day brings, to remain in conscious
contact with the spiritual principles of my recovery. The more I
do this, the more balance I have, and the better equipped I am to
accept the full range of experience that life has to offer, and I do so
with patience, courage, and love.

*I understand that practicing principles means applying patience,
tolerance, acceptance, and humility in my life while I wait for
things to work out.*

27

KINDNESS

"Sometimes kindness is a sincere, well-timed smile of support. Other times, it requires our effort to be present and silent when words are not adequate or it asks us to empathize with or support another."
Of Character: Building Assets in Recovery

When I'm in emotional distress it's particularly difficult to even extend a smile to another person. I get stuck in the toxic mindset of "if they only knew," or "they don't understand my pain," or any number of other self-pitying, toxic shame statements that continue to separate me from others. Separation leads to distance, distance to isolation, and isolation to actively addictive behaviors. This behavior leads to the abuse of medication. Kindness is the bridge between myself and others. It is particularly important to extend that bridge, that lifeline, to others when I'm feeling emotions that are painful, fearful, angry, shameful, guilty, or lonely. In active addiction, I used manipulation and character defects to draw people in. In pain recovery, I do it with a smile, a warm embrace, a close connection with another human being. Through kindness, I'm connected. Through connection, I'm freed from active addiction.

I smile at others, especially when I'm feeling emotions that would normally cause me not to smile. I extend a special type of kindness to others, knowing that my recovery depends on my connection with others. My emotional balance depends on kindness to others.

HOPE

PHYSICAL BALANCE

···

"It is believed that chronic pain
is one of the most common causes of suicide."
A Day without Pain

The general public may not necessarily appreciate or respect
chronic pain for the problem that it really is, but that does not stand
in the way of my recovery. I do not need other people to understand
the depth of the pain (only part of which is physical). Instead, I
focus more on understanding my own problem, seeking more to
understand my pain, appreciate that it is part of me, and know that
I do not need to be a statistic who falls victim, paying the ultimate
price for physical suffering. I can focus on the solution with a
healthy appreciation for the scope of the problem, never forgetting
what it is that I'm up against and what it must require in recovery.
I can also understand and reach out to others who may have yet to
experience the freedom I've found in recovery, remembering what
they are up against, as well as how difficult it is to get through that
first day, week, or month without medication.

*I remember the true depth and scope of my addiction and chronic pain
and their consequences, knowing that I must commit to my recovery—
it being truly a matter of life and death.*

THOUGHTS TO ACTIONS, POSITIVE ACTION

MENTAL BALANCE

"The process of moving from sensing and thinking to taking action usually happens almost instantaneously. I remember that while it feels that way, it is actually a multi-step process. I take the time to remember how this process is unique for me but includes six steps: sensory perceptions, thoughts, feelings, wants and needs, identifying and considering options, then taking action.

When my thinking is healthy and balanced I progress through the six steps on a continuous basis and almost unconsciously.... In pain recovery I can handle the feelings that come up so that I can really identify what I want and need."

Adapted from Pain Recovery: How to Find Balance
and Reduce Suffering from Chronic Pain

My recovery is serious business, but I remember not to take myself so seriously, and I remain calm; the right thoughts and actions become apparent if I remain calm and have faith in the process. Soon, I will be moving almost seamlessly from right thoughts to right actions, and I remember that what works for others can work for me, too.

I consciously slow down my thought process today, thinking of my brain as a muscle and making sure that I'm taking each step during the process. Pain recovery is about constantly exercising that muscle to think differently, taking the time to remember my feelings, wants, needs, and options before acting.

SHAME AND GUILT

EMOTIONAL BALANCE

....

"Guilt is an emotion wherein I feel that I've made a
mistake. It is defined as a feeling of having committed
some wrong or failed in an obligation. Shame, on the
other hand, is an emotion wherein the feeling is that
I am a mistake. Shame is defined as a painful feeling
of humiliation or distress that may be caused by the
conscious awareness of wrong or foolish behavior.
Often it is not even attached to a specific behavior, but
to how I perceive myself internally. These two feelings
often exist in partnership for people with chronic pain."
Adapted from Pain Recovery: How to Find Balance
and Reduce Suffering from Chronic Pain

The emotional experience of shame is based on a belief that there's
something intrinsically wrong with me as a person. Deep inside
I feel fundamentally flawed, and believe that everyone knows it.
Having chronic pain feeds into and strengthens this belief. It can
be difficult to escape from the burden of shame I have internalized
as a result of the life experiences I may have had before and during
my active addiction. When I'm shame-based, anything I do that is
less than perfect reinforces my belief that I'm defective, and
that I have been all along.

*I am kinder in my estimate of myself than I used to be. Today
I feel good about my character assets—they do exist. I need not live
in shame; I am no better and no worse than anyone else. What a
gift to myself that realization is.*

LACK OF FAITH
SPIRITUAL BALANCE

....

"Fear ends when faith begins."
Unknown

Fear is the overwhelming concern, the debilitating concern about what others think. Fear is the incessant preoccupation with the idea that some*thing*, some*one*, or some*place* might hurt me.

Faith, on the other hand, consists of having those fears, but taking action anyway. Faith to me means taking the appropriate action in my life and leaving the results to my God/Spirit/higher power. The feelings of fear and faith can exist at the same time. The actions related to fear and faith cancel each other out—I'm either acting out my fear or acting out my faith at any given moment. When I'm acting out my fear I have a lack of faith; the action of faith is the action of putting one foot in front of the other despite my doubt or fear.

I have faith in recovery and the process by taking action for my recovery regardless of how I'm feeling and leaving the results to my God/Spirit/higher power.

Thurs. night
<u>10</u> Benefit (art's) PAIN
Bring letter FROM PAIN   Friday 5·25·17
to me.
DR MUEHLLER
"frantically honest..."

e nothing.

Narrative therapy
        How We Tell Our Story
(ies...)